The Pursuit of Hope

*A Pulitzer Prize winner
tells the story of how she
and many others fought
—and conquered—the fear, uncertainty,
and despair of multiple sclerosis*

ALSO BY MIRIAM OTTENBERG
The Federal Investigators

The Pursuit of Hope

by Miriam Ottenberg

Foreword by Dr. DONALD B. TOWER,
National Institutes of Health

RAWSON, WADE PUBLISHERS, INC.
NEW YORK

Library of Congress Cataloging in Publication Data

Ottenberg, Miriam.
 The pursuit of hope.

 Includes index.
 1.   Multiple sclerosis—Biography.   2.   Ottenberg,
Miriam.   I.   Title.
RC377.O87   1978   362.1'9'683409   78–54041
ISBN 0–89256–069–X

Published simultaneously in Canada by
McClelland and Stewart, Ltd.

Manufactured in the United States of America
by The Book Press, Brattleboro, Vermont

Designed by A. Christopher Simon

FIFTH PRINTING MAY 1979

Foreword

The pathological characteristics of multiple sclerosis (MS) were first depicted in drawings of brain and spinal cord specimens published by Hooper, Cruveilhier, and Carswell nearly 150 years ago. But it was not until 1868 that the great French neurologist Jean-Martin Charcot, working at the famous Salpêtrière hospital in Paris, named the process *sclérose en plaques* and described the complete symptomatology and pathology of MS, differentiating it from other disorders, such as Parkinson's disease.

Over the century since Charcot's clinical studies the enigma of MS has defied countless dedicated investigators. In a recent extensive review of the current status of MS research (*Science* 195:969, 1977), it was concluded that multiple sclerosis is an exceptionally complicated disorder, resulting from complex interactions of genetic, environmental, geographic, viral, and immunologic factors. Despite the progress being made in understanding these individual components, no clear picture of the entire process, and hence no definitive therapy, emerges.

Both of the major MS funding agencies in the United States —the federal National Institute of Neurological and Communicative Disorders and Stroke (NINCDS) and the private National Multiple Sclerosis Society—have intensified the research assault on MS with the expectation that breakthroughs in any one of these areas will provide means of halting the spread of the disorder and of alleviating its symptoms. Meanwhile for the millions of MS patients around the world, the battle continues against the constant challenges that this disorder poses to their daily lives.

Multiple sclerosis is a lifelong disorder whose unpredictable and often chaotic nature can dishearten even the most stalwart of its victims. In this sensitive, informative and compelling book, Miriam Ottenberg captures and clarifies the disorder's profound physical and emotional effects. At the same time, she offers hope through the encouraging examples of patients whose ingenious and positive combating of their problems brings a sense of order, cohesion, and fulfillment into their lives.

Few endeavors hold more promise for MS victims than the vigorous work of basic medical researchers. Miriam Ottenberg's description of the MS research assault serves her readers well; she strikes an appropriate balance between the excitement of new research leads and the cautious judgment required to think in terms of advances rather than miraculous breakthroughs.

MS patients, their families, and friends will find much to encourage them in these pages. Health-care practitioners who treat and help MS victims will also learn much from Miriam Ottenberg's work. The intimate confidences of the men and women she has interviewed enable us to better understand their fears, misconceptions, and needs, to share their world, and to join them in the pursuit of hope.

DONALD B. TOWER, M.D., Ph.D.

Director
National Institute of Neurological
and Communicative Disorders and Stroke
National Institutes of Health
Bethesda, Maryland

Preface

Many patients with multiple sclerosis made this book possible. They come from as far away as New Zealand and as near as the apartment next door. They are black and white, working and retired, some just out of school, some entering middle age. Single, married, widowed . . . they run the gamut of living arrangements.

Different in so many ways, they have two things in common. All knew by now that the bizarre symptoms they experienced were due to multiple sclerosis. And all of them were so intent on helping others understand this mysterious ailment that they were willing to let me use their names in this book. Every name here is the name of a real person with a real experience. For many years, young men and women, and more especially their relatives, made multiple sclerosis a "closet disease" under the mistaken idea that some stigma attached to it. With this book, they are telling the world that they have a neurological disease that could happen to any young person until science discovers a way to stop it. Wholeheartedly, my MS friends have joined in my pursuit of hope, and I thank all of them.

If it had not been for I. William Hill, my long-time boss at *The Washington Star*, I would never have met them. I have him to thank for launching me on my quest and suggesting the book.

My thanks are due also to leaders in multiple sclerosis research who have given so generously of their time and knowledge to make this book accurate as well as informative. I owe special thanks to Dr. John F. Kurtzke, chief of the neurology service at the Veterans Administration Hospital in Washington and professor of neurology at Georgetown University School of Medicine; Dr. Guy McKhann, professor of neurology at Johns Hopkins Medical Institutions; Dr. William E. Reynolds, deputy director of research programs, National Multiple Sclerosis Society; Dr. Dale E. McFarlin, chief, and Dr. Henry F. McFarland, assistant chief, Neuroimmunology Branch, National Institute of Neurological and Communicative Disorders and Stroke (NINCDS); Dr. Wallace W. Tourtellotte, chief of the neurology service at the Veterans Administration's Wadsworth Hospital Center in Los Angeles; and Dr. James Q. Simmons, former director of medical programs, National Multiple Sclerosis Society.

I am especially grateful to Sylvia Lawry, founder and executive director of the National Multiple Sclerosis Society, not only for telling me the painful details of her early efforts to get her brother's illness diagnosed but also for making sure that her staff gave me the fullest cooperation in my search for facts.

My gratitude likewise goes to Diane Afes, director of patient services, National Capital Chapter of the National Multiple Sclerosis Society, who arranged interviews with MS patients, took me to rap sessions with them, organized the yoga classes I had suggested, and endlessly interpreted the emotional problems and needs of the people to whom she shows such devotion.

Dr. Donald B. Tower, director of the National Institute of Neurological and Communicative Disorders and Stroke, offered "help in every way we possibly can" and certainly made

good on that promise, particularly through the continuing
assistance given by Carolyn Holstein, science writer for
NINCDS. My thanks go, too, to Jeannette Hopkins, the editor
who kept the book on track and on deadline.

Washington, D.C., April 1978   MIRIAM OTTENBERG

Contents

The Pursuit of Hope

Chapter 1

Beginning the Pursuit of Hope

One week in May 1960, I won the Pulitzer Prize, for exposing used-car frauds, and lost my father. He and mother had been traveling overseas. The night they heard I had won they called to congratulate me, but the next night the international operator woke me at 3:00 A.M. and mother told me my father had just died of a cerebral hemorrhage. About a week later I started across the street and a policeman jerked me back to the curb.

"That car was nearly on top of you," he scolded. "Why don't you look where you're going?"

Too shaken to speak, I could not tell him the car appeared to me to be half a block away. Certainly, I would not admit that all the cars now stopped for a light looked like those two-layered, over-the-road car haulers. I did not know then, would not know for many years, that I had temporarily lost my depth perception, that the two-layered look of the cars was a mirage created by double vision, and that the cause of it was multiple sclerosis.

I know now that many believe the shock of sudden death can trigger an attack of a disease so mysterious that half a million people in this country and many thousands more in other lands who have it or a closely related illness never know what the next day may do to them.

In the 1960s, though, I had never heard of multiple sclerosis. Why should I? It had nothing to do with me—or so I thought. My doctor knew differently, but he decided not to tell me, and, for me, I think the decision was right at the time. If I had known, I might have turned cautious. I might not have trusted my legs to take me into danger and out again, might not have ventured into Mau Mau country or into Malaya when guerrillas were shooting up the countryside, might not have posed as the willing dupe of con men for my stories for *The Washington Star*.

For the hundred or more friends with multiple sclerosis I have accumulated in the past two years, however, not knowing what was wrong with them just made them worse. They had a need to know the cause of their bizarre symptoms, usually much more terrifying than mine. I was too busy trying to uncover organized crime, corruption, and a remarkable variety of consumer frauds to wonder why I fell so much. Even when I tripped over a slight bump in the newsroom floor and shattered my elbow, I was too involved with trying to wind up an exposé of condominium shortcomings from my hospital bed to speculate about why I tripped.

Six years after my father's death, I told my doctor, just in fun, "My housekeeper says if you were any kind of a doctor, you would find out why I fall all the time."

He looked over my medical record. "Do you fall much?" "Pretty often," I admitted, wishing I had kept my mouth shut because he looked so serious. He asked me to wait outside, and a few minutes later he emerged with his coat on and an ultimatum.

"I'm taking you to the hospital," he said. "Your housekeeper will bring you your things."

In vain, I protested all the way to the car that I had an investigation to complete before the weekend. For days, I was bled and stabbed and tapped. Between times, I would call my bad-guy targets for my stories and impersonate a beleaguered housewife—to the wide-eyed amazement of the three other patients in the room. Robert Kennedy sent me a delicate basket of flowers. His exploits in fighting organized crime had kept me on page one of *The Washington Star* for years. His rose buds were the only cheerful moment in several anxious days.

The verdict was "a demyelinating disease"—familiar words to patients with multiple sclerosis, totally unfamiliar to me. Years later, when I asked my doctor why he hadn't said multiple sclerosis instead of a demyelinating disease, he retorted, "You're a reporter. I thought you'd look it up."

Now I know that a sheath of fatty tissue, called myelin, insulates the brain and spinal cord of the central nervous system. As telephone calls go astray when the insulation frays, so the messages from the brain are slowed, misdirected, or lost entirely when even a pinpoint of myelin is damaged or "demyelinated."

All that I learned much later, when I made the connection between demyelination and multiple sclerosis. That happened —as it has happened with so many of my new friends—because I was listening to a ball game and an athlete came on to urge contributions for research into a disease that crippled. He said it may strike arms, legs, eyes, bladder, and balance and that nobody knows what causes it or how to cure it. The symptoms sounded familiar. I called my doctor.

"Hey," I asked with my usual aplomb, "do I have multiple sclerosis?"

Long pause, then, "I told you that long ago." But he never had. My own blinders had been firmly in place for years.

Much later, as I faced the doctor then in charge of the *Star*'s medical clinic, I learned that I was being retired on disability. The falls were coming oftener. Right in the middle of a major investigation, I had fallen and cracked my knee.

The newspaper business, I told myself now, had given me glory enough for two lifetimes and I should be ready to leave the investigating to someone else and begin a new career. "I'll keep on working at home," I told the doctor confidently. His long face seemed to grow longer. "Work?" he said doubtfully. "But not for long."

When the impact of his words hit me, the walls of his office seemed to close in. The voice of doom frightened me. Then anger pushed out fear.

"That's a terrible thing to say. You won't stop me, but you could destroy a person's hope with that kind of talk."

His look of patient pity stopped my outburst. I wanted to escape from that office, and I did, but I could not escape his words. Was multiple sclerosis that devastating? I could not believe I was through.

My newspaper friends gave me an electric typewriter as a retirement present, at least *they* thought I could go on working. Then I had a chilling thought: They did not know I had multiple sclerosis. Only the doctors knew—or suspected. I had kept the diagnosis a secret for fear someone would tell my then eighty-eight-year-old mother. All she knew about multiple sclerosis was the sight of her brother's wife, Aunt Sara, in a wheelchair. I did not want her lively imagination to put me there, too. As far as she knew, I was retiring early because my car pool had retired, and taking six buses to work and back was getting me down. She did not need to know and I did not tell her. (Yes, she has to know now, three years later, but as the book goes to press, I am still trying to figure out the best way to tell her.)*

---

* I have told her. Turns out she is relieved to know that the way she broke the news of my father's death had nothing to do with my limp. She had that secret feeling of guilt all these years. Now I am aware of the value of open communications.

My own verdict seemed more pressing than the verdicts in nineteenth-century murders I had planned to write a book about. If a diagnosis of multiple sclerosis was tantamount to a death sentence, why hadn't I died long ago? I had had the same symptoms for a number of years. If it sentenced victims to life in a wheelchair, as I had heard, I wouldn't still be walking around—limping, but on my own two feet. I wouldn't have been able to break the story of Joe Valachi, Cosa Nostra, and the Godfather; I would not have sought the islands of the world from Zanzibar to Tasmania.

There had to be answers that gloomy doctor did not know. For at least some of us—maybe most of us—there had to be hope. I would defy him, prove him wrong—him and all crepe hangers who thought of multiple sclerosis as doom.

I would become a reporter again. I would investigate multiple sclerosis the way I had investigated home-improvement frauds and get-rich-quick swindles. I'd go to the prime source —the victims. I'd talk to men and women with multiple sclerosis, their husbands and wives, their families and friends. If there were heroes, I'd find them. If there were villains, I'd uncover them. I would try to find out how my victims weathered their disease, and especially what could give them hope.

The adrenaline of the investigative reporter was flowing again. I opened the door deliberately kept shut and locked in my mind and heart for so long—the door to multiple sclerosis.

From the start, I was confident—as I am now with more reason—that all the money the National Multiple Sclerosis Society and the government are spending to find what causes the disease and how it can be cured will pay off in the next ten years, maybe sooner. My quest, however, was more urgent. Mine was the pursuit of hope now.

As an old friend was to say later, everybody knows somebody with multiple sclerosis (one reason why I think the figure of half a million is badly understated). It was my mother who inadvertently provided my first victim. One day, she came into my apartment in a great state of agitation to say her young friend, Lois Ryan, had multiple sclerosis. I knew she was picturing Lois in a wheelchair like Aunt Sara—as she would picture me if I were to tell her. I kept my face expressionless as mother went on. "Do you remember telling me once that Sara would have benefited from yoga exercises? If Lois's doctor approves, can you get Lois in your yoga class?"

Driving back and forth to our yoga class, I questioned Lois about her disease. For weeks I asked questions and she gave answers that shook me more than she could know. Finally, I blurted out, "I've got MS too, but don't tell mother." It was to become for me a constant refrain. For my victims to talk freely, I had to join them. No impersonation this time. I wanted them to know they were not alone as some of them seemed to feel, that there are a lot of us out there, learning to cope, reaching out for hope.

Lois steered me to the National Multiple Sclerosis Society. I did not know that the society has more than two hundred chapters, branches, clinics, centers across the country not only raising money for research but caring for patients, bringing them together to talk out mutual problems, supplying wheelchairs and aids to daily living, combing the resources of a city for anything that would make life easier, providing professional help and counseling, and literature.

Over the two years of my quest for hope, I watched one chapter in action almost daily as I became successively investigative reporter, mother confessor to my victims, their friend, and, finally, crusader.

At the beginning, though, all I cared about was a source of victims for my story and the National Capital chapter was a natural because Washington is a city of transients, people from someplace else ultimately going someplace else. I could get a cross-section of the population without ever leaving town.

The society's patient-services director started me off with a shock, though, by suggesting that I interview Gerald Shur, the Justice Department official in charge of providing new identities to keep "hit men" away from those willing to testify against the Mafia or Cosa Nostra. I had known him years ago when both of us were involved in Kennedy's war on organized crime.

I was almost afraid to open Shur's door, afraid of what I would find. I need not have worried. He looked and behaved as he always had—smiling, friendly, helpful. After we had gotten past the "I had no idea you had it, too," business, we began to talk. For a moment there, I felt like the walking wounded meeting on a battlefield in no man's land, uncertain where the bullets were coming from or where they might hit next.

His onslaught had begun quite suddenly when he was thirty-three. He had dismissed "funny little things that happened" earlier as nothing more than working too hard. But that night, as his wife was watching TV and he was reading, suddenly he began to feel nauseated. He couldn't see very well. He tried to stand and found he couldn't. He put his arms around his wife, and she said, "Your eyes are crossed."

At first he thought he had had a stroke. "I had pins and needles in my arms. I couldn't understand what was happening to me. I was absolutely terrified, absolutely sure I was going to die. The only comfort was my wife holding my hand. She stayed at the hospital all day, all night, all the next day. It was a Catholic hospital with a crucifix in the room. When I opened my eyes, I saw four Jesuses, instead of one. Me, a good Jewish boy!"

We could share a laugh now at his quadruple vision. More than a decade later, his sight is clear and he is walking and working every day. We began to swap symptoms like matching battle scars. I said his quadruple vision beat my double vision of a few years back, but I bet he had experienced nothing like what I called my jigsaw-puzzle vision.

"I was interviewing the police chief," I recalled, "and all at once, his face had no nose. Then an eye disappeared and the nose came back. It was like looking at a jigsaw puzzle with half the pieces missing. An ophthalmologist said I was having muscle spasm behind the eyes. He was supposed to be the best eye man in town, but he missed this one." When I was interviewing a neurologist recently, I told Shur, he recognized my long gone jigsaw-puzzle vision immediately as optic neuritis, often the first indication of multiple sclerosis. I liked his description better than mine. He called it "an island of darkness in a sea of vision." The medical name is scotoma.

Until Gerry Shur got multiple sclerosis he didn't know anybody else with the disease. "Now I keep running into it. A deputy marshal assigned to my office has it. There's a lawyer in the civil division and the man who teaches the band at my son's school. This fellow was staggering around so much that one day the janitor winked at him and said, 'I wish I had some of what you have.' The bandmaster did a double take before he realized the janitor thought he was drunk." He confided to Shur that he had mentioned his illness to no one because he thought it carried a stigma like a social disease. "My God," said Shur, "you don't even have the same fun getting it!"

In a few minutes, Shur had capsuled the fear, the uncertainty, even the needless shame sometimes experienced by people with our disease. He himself had slid all the way down, believing he had gone to the hospital to die and coming home to a sense of hopeless desolation. Now he was back doing an important job at Justice, his sense of humor even sharper than I remembered. He had shared his hope with me.

Since then, the pursuit of hope has brought me the music of folk singer-author-environmentalist Gary Smith, who was a park ranger until multiple sclerosis ended his mountain climbing. I watched Robert Douglas, a former virologist driven from his test tubes by the disease, teaching a blind child how to jump her horse. I lunched with newlyweds to hear about their wheelchair wedding. Love and marriage were important questions to which I needed answers. I listened to the travel story of a fellow journalist from New Zealand, who started out with a cane, wound up in a wheelchair, but managed a 30,000-mile world trip. A Buffalo prosecutor described how he dragged his crippled legs through the city's worst blizzard to reach court for a murder trial—only to find half the jurors had failed to show up. I learned how Dr. Joseph J. Panzarella, Jr., earned White House recognition as 1977 Handicapped American of the Year, and met the wife who made it possible for him to carry six jobs at once despite his inability to move anything but his head. I watched a Multiple Sclerosis Mother of the Year, Barbara McGrath, serving the gourmet meal she had cooked herself, and remembered her description of playing the Good Fairy in a performance of *The Wizard of Oz* at her sons' school, her wheelchair concealed under the Good Fairy's crinoline. In the narrow lobby of a convalescent hospital, Eliza Ann Dobson sang me a spiritual she had composed and sold to raise $500 for multiple sclerosis research. An old newspaper friend, Eileen Shanahan, who left her job on the *New York Times* to become assistant secretary of the Department of Health, Education and Welfare for public affairs, introduced me to her psychiatrist sister. Dr. Kathleen Shanahan Cohen had been named New Jersey Medical Woman of the Year despite the leg brace she conceals under her pants suit.

As word got around that I was seeking what I could only call victims, because that was how I had always tagged the people I interviewed in newspaper days, tips kept coming. The administrator of my insurance program led me to Alma Gaghan, who raised seven children despite multiple sclerosis. The nurse in my doctor's office told me to call her friend Penny

Renzi, whose military husband keeps her life on an even keel.

I was not looking for Pollyanna yarns and did not get them. One woman admitted her husband beat her. A girl described how she crawled across a hospital parking lot, the gravel tearing at her knees, because she had no one to drive her to the hospital. A young wife confided: "My mother-in-law says I cheated her son." They talked to me because I was one of them, sometimes because they were more lonely than healthy people could ever be, but more often because they too were pursuing hope. They knew I had to hear the experiences that pulled them down, along with their upbeat moments. How else could I uncover the despoilers, the careless or callous destroyers of hope?

The first person who actively refused to let the despoilers of hope beat her down told me her story, too. Sylvia Lawry, the founder and still executive director of the National Multiple Sclerosis Society, the moving spirit in forming the International Federation of Multiple Sclerosis Societies, started a pursuit of hope to help her younger brother when she was twenty-one years old.

I followed the traditional pattern of the investigative reporter—from the victims to the authorities with possible answers. My quest led me to the National Institute of Neurological and Communicative Disorders and Stroke (NINCDS), to the National Multiple Sclerosis Society, to a Veterans Administration Hospital as I asked scientists and physicians what they are doing to discover the cause of multiple sclerosis and how they can treat it before they have a cure.

Multiple sclerosis, I discovered, is now considered the most common disease of the central nervous system, more prevalent than ALS (amyotrophic lateral sclerosis, or Lou Gehrig's disease) and more common than muscular dystrophy, which every person with multiple sclerosis knows is often confused with it. Since nobody knows for sure just how widespread it really is—some people with the disease are too timid to admit they have it even to the society set up to help them—NINCDS has undertaken a survey of the country's neurologists and neurosurgeons and approximately two thousand general practitioners (selected at random). They are being asked to identify all possible and probable multiple sclerosis patients seen through the years. Hospitals also are being surveyed to pin down how many cases they have had. Some patients are keeping a ninety-day diary of all health-related expenditures to find out what the disease costs them and their families directly as well as indirectly, the wages they have lost as well as the wages lost by whoever in the family may stay home to look after them. Nationwide, the cost of multiple sclerosis has been estimated at $2 billion, but that may be as underestimated as the size of the multiple sclerosis population.

The disease that costs so much to so many has been around for a century and a half. In some ways, I learned right at the start of my investigation, we are still no wiser than was Count Augustus D'Este, a young English nobleman who recorded in his 1822 diary that he had fallen victim to a mysterious disease. While D'Este, like so many others after him, searched all over Europe for a cure that failed to materialize, a British medical illustrator named Sir Robert Carswell included in his *Pathological Anatomy* (1838) a watercolor of a spinal cord marred by spots of hardened or discolored tissue. About the same time, a French physician, Jean Cruveilhier, saw similar spots on the spinal cord of a long-hospitalized woman at autopsy. He called the spots islands of sclerosis (from the Greek word for "hardening") and speculated that those spots might have caused her illness.

There speculation about the mysterious ailment rested until 1868, when Jean-Martin Charcot, the great French medical investigator, gave the disease not only a name but its first detailed description. Charcot had found that many of his patients at the Salpêtrière Hospital in Paris suffered from tremors, jerky movements, and varied degrees of paralysis that fitted no disease identified at that time. At autopsy, he noticed plaques or hardened patches throughout the central nervous system. He called the disease *sclérose en plaques*. Because of the varied locations of these patches, the British called the disease disseminated sclerosis. Americans named it multiple sclerosis.

The location of these patches—the places in the brain and spinal cord where the insulation over the nerve fibers sloughs off—determines what body functions are affected. When nerve impulses that normally race through the central nervous system at a 225-mile-an-hour clip are slowed to maybe a tenth that speed, the eyes may lose their sight or half their field of vision; the fingers may get too numb to hold a pencil; the bladder may lose control; or the legs may stiffen. You could have a pinpoint of demyelination in the frontal lobes and never have reason to believe anything is amiss. An identical lesion somewhere else in the body could cause all hell to break loose. That's why no two multiple sclerosis patients look alike or experience the same symptoms, although they have the same disease. Not only does their disease not follow the same course but even the same person will look and feel different with every episode.

The very nature of multiple sclerosis, its roller-coaster pattern of exacerbations and remissions, the storms and calms of the disease, set a trap for the unwary doctor. He or she never know—or did not know until very recently—whether treatment actually helped the patient or whether the patient would have done just as well with only compassion and caring.

Just as there is no certain treatment, there is yet no cure. The ongoing medical detective work centers on finding the cause. In the course of that search, they have discovered enough to raise questions that challenge the investigator.

Why are more young people stricken in Michigan than Missouri, in Wales than Italy, and in the Shetland and Orkney islands more often than anywhere else?

How does it happen that hot weather, too much concentrated sunshine, can bring on an attack, but the closer one gets to the equator, the less of the disease one finds?

Why does it surface for the first time usually between the ages of twenty and forty, rarely before eighteen or after forty-five?

What makes it so variable that a person can have the disease and never know it or suffer such a direct hit that the future means a wheelchair or even a life in bed?

Why does it strike more women than men, more college graduates than grade-school dropouts, the middle- rather than the lower-income group, more whites than blacks?

Those unanswered questions actually put me on the road to hope. Ten years ago, sometimes later than that, researchers lacked enough facts even to pose the questions. Certainly that is progress.

Nearly three years have passed since Gerry Shur and I swapped symptoms and I began forming my unanswered questions. I sensed then that my pursuit of hope was headed in the right direction. Now, I am sure of it.

Chapter 2

Exploring the Mystery Illness

Without warning, Barbara McGrath collapsed on the bathroom floor. Frightened and helpless, she screamed to her husband in the motel bedroom. "George, help me! I can't get up."

All the wedding to-do—the excitement of getting married, the strain of greeting two hundred and fifty guests at the reception, the rush to get off on the honeymoon—had combined to trigger an attack of the disease that would ultimately put Barbara into a wheelchair. She had multiple sclerosis but did not know it, would not know it for many months. The motel doctor smiled comfortably as he told her to take it easy. "Just honeymoon nerves." Barbara sensed it was more than that. Six years earlier when she was a young buyer for a Washington department store, her legs also had felt shaky, and friends told her she was not walking straight. A doctor suggested she sleep on the floor, and she and her roommate dutifully hauled their mattress off the bed every night. When she went home to find out what was wrong, her parents had to help her off the airplane at New Haven. The doctors gave her many tests but few answers. After a three-month rest she felt well enough to go off to Europe to visit the Pope, ski, dance, and play for four carefree months.

By the time she met George McGrath at the Army-Navy Club in Washington, on New Year's Day 1961, six years had passed. She had visited a doctor only once in those years, when her vision blurred and she was seeing double. The doctor found nothing wrong and after a while, her eyes returned to normal. Nobody connected the hurting, buckling legs and the double vision. At least, nobody mentioned it to Barbara. When she visited her family doctor for premarital tests and he inquired how she was getting along, she beamed, "Just fine," and he advised her, "Don't get overtired, don't overdo." She was still unaware that her family doctor suspected something might be seriously wrong.

Facing me now across the living room she had decorated herself, looking younger than her years, as most women with multiple sclerosis seem to do, Barbara went back to the tumble during the honeymoon. "When we came home and my legs were still bothering me, we saw a doctor. He said I was pregnant. I was so happy. But, I told him, I had the same feeling I had in my legs years ago. So he sent me to another doctor and I was put in the hospital. George tells me now that the doctor said I had multiple sclerosis then but that I was not to be told, and George didn't tell me.

"I was being pushed along by an attendant on my way to therapy, and since I'll read anything in front of me, I opened this little steel folder on my lap and started to read. It was my medical record, and I remember it saying, *The patient is completely unaware of the seriousness of her condition.* The report said I was gregarious, happy, and they didn't know how to tell me about my condition. I kept on reading. Finally, it said, *We think we shall tell the patient tomorrow morning that she has multiple sclerosis.*

"I asked the therapist, 'Do you know I have multiple sclerosis?' She looked startled. 'It says here you're not supposed to know.' By the time the doctor arrived, I was crushed, in tears.

My whole life was turning around and I didn't know how to accept it."

Barbara McGrath made such a good job of accepting it that she became Multiple Sclerosis Mother of the Year and filled a scrapbook for her two sons with stories of the honors that have come her way.

If emotional shock is enough to trigger an attack, however, the careless way she learned the truth was enough to slow her recovery.

Nobody, neither physician nor researcher, knows why multiple sclerosis strikes or what causes this long-slumbering disease to surface and resurface. In Barbara McGrath's case, the disease probably emerged first when she was twenty-three and overworking. The emotional stress surrounding her wedding could have triggered the next episode. Multiple sclerosis acts that way, sometimes coming on so strong that the patient has to be rushed to the hospital, other times insinuating itself into a victim's life so slyly that the first time or two it is no more than a puzzling discomfort. After a week or a month, it may disappear to return a year or five years later or never again. Sometimes, it comes and never leaves, progressing slowly or—in a minority of cases—swiftly to a wheelchair life or even a life in bed. It is the most common disease of the central nervous system and the most unpredictable.

It can paralyze the legs or stiffen them to a staggering walk. It can blind, at least temporarily or in only one eye, or leave a victim color blind. It can send shock waves racing down the spine or force a person to stutter or slur words. It can make legs so cold that, as Donna Matzureff put it, she was sure she could chill a pail of beer just by putting her leg in it. Or the legs can feel so flaming hot that Elaine Dewar cut off her jeans above the knees in a Connecticut winter because she could not bear the touch of cloth against her burning skin. The frequently bizarre sensations are hard enough to take when the person knows he has multiple sclerosis. When somebody has never even heard of the disease and suddenly sees two lines dividing the highway when he knows there should be only one, he can panic.

Recognizing the symptoms of multiple sclerosis could be the first step on the road to hope. A man needs to know he is not losing his mind when he walks across the room with a pen in his hand and finds his hand empty when he starts to write. Or steps out of his slippers without being aware of it. The pen dropped from his hand because his fingers were numb and he walked out of his slippers because he had lost feeling in his feet. No matter how odd his sensations, he is not going crazy, as he might fear.

Understanding symptoms, particularly invisible ones, is important, too, for husbands and wives and other relatives of victims because otherwise they are inclined to wonder—frequently aloud—whether anything is really wrong. That also goes for friends who ask why old Fred, their drinking buddy, has turned into a party poop.

Marilyn Pollin, a psychiatric social worker, suspected she was losing her mind when milk bottles slipped through her fingers to crash on the kitchen floor. Jewell Phillips was twice sent home from a hospital emergency room with tranquilizers before she was finally admitted for treatment—and even then, she was put on the psychiatric ward. One woman who progressively deteriorated over two years was told by one doctor after another that her problem was "anxiety hysteria."

A victim who knows others with the disease often must cope with a pressing fear: Am I going to be like that? Alma Gaghan could only think of the man down the block whose children went to school with her children. "I didn't know what MS was until it hit this man. I didn't see him for a while, and when he reappeared he was blind and his legs were in braces. I got a chill at the sight of him, just thinking, *O my God, he's so young*. Now I was told I had multiple sclerosis."

When mother's friend Lois learned she had multiple sclerosis she could think only of the husband of a woman in her office, "a miserable man who couldn't do anything for himself, not even turn over in bed." Dr. Frank Uhlmann, former chief psychologist of the Labor Department and now consulting psychologist of several government agencies, told me he was "more uptight" about his diagnosis because the wife of his college roommate had it—"within six months she was confined to a wheelchair, six months later she was almost a vegetable, and in another six months she was dead."

Lois, Alma, and Frank learned their diagnoses years ago. All are still working at least part of every day, enjoying their children, at last convinced that they are not going the way of the first victims they knew and that not all victims of multiple sclerosis are alike.

The majority of patients I have met had gone through years, even decades, of fleeting symptoms that perplexed before they alarmed. Who but a full-blown hypochondriac rushes to the doctor because a hand prickles with pins and needles or a foot drags when she is tired or she has this overwhelming desire for naps? A good night's sleep may be all a body needs to feel fine again. When my eyes started acting up and my legs suddenly buckled and I fell, I would explain: "When God thinks I'm working too hard, He'll hit the only two parts of me that can slow a reporter down—the eyes or the legs." That was my way of brushing off symptoms, even when my doctor ordered me to bed for a week.

When Mildred Smith cut her arm on a hoe, had a tetanus shot, and soon afterward went blind, she remembered reading about a woman temporarily blinded after a tetanus shot. She simply waited for her sight to return and it finally did. When Dr. Kathleen Shanahan Cohen, moonlighting on an overcrowded maternity ward during her last year in medical school, was overcome by such severe cramps that interns lifted her onto a stretcher and gave her painkillers, she shrugged it off as the penalty of trying to do too much. When Tony Rodolakis, a "think tank" expert turned stockbroker, opened his eyes to an oddly twisted ceiling and the room whirled as he tried to get out of bed, he blamed it on a bad hangover, even though he had had little to drink the night before. An incident on the way to work scared him. "It was a cold, clear December day," Tony recalled, "but when I hit a straight stretch of road, there was this ground fog for maybe a hundred yards. My newly disoriented vision totally confused me and I almost panicked. I inched along until I broke out of the fog, and when I got to work I felt so dizzy I thought I'd better see a doctor." The doctor treated Tony for a middle-ear infection. When the dizziness passed in a few weeks, Tony assumed the doctor had been right—assumed it, that is, until six months later when he was playing tennis with his brother and saw two balls, three balls. His brother had never beaten him at tennis before, and it started Tony on his long quest for the cause of his problem.

People have trouble explaining what bothers them. "I feel like a fool," Donna Matzureff told her doctor, "but my hand seems to close into a claw and I put my hand under my pillow at night to try to straighten it out." Elaine Dewar tried and failed to explain that her arm seemed to be curling up. She had no better success making a doctor understand that she felt her spine was vibrating, that she was shaking like a leaf when he could see she was not shaking at all. How explain what Eliza Dobson meant when she said, "My feet got stubborn on the floor," or what Marilyn Pollin was going through when she described the sensation of a boa constrictor wrapped around her legs, or what a man at a rap session meant when he said his face was falling in?

Because symptoms seem so bizarre or lend themselves to such bizarre descriptions, physicians may either refuse to believe anything is wrong or reach for an understandable diagnosis. When a forty-year-old woman told her family doctor her legs had gotten so stiff she could no longer stoop to put food in the oven, he told her, "You know, you're not getting any younger." When Penny Renzi tried to find out why her vision had become so blurred she was afraid to drive, an eye specialist told her she had a hive in the retina, which, he said, happened to the elderly and heavy smokers. Penny was a twenty-year-old nonsmoker.

Maladies that later can be traced to early signs of multiple sclerosis are diagnosed at the time as high or low blood pressure, a high cholesterol count, poor circulation, diabetes, a slipped disc, a thyroid deficiency, side effects of pregnancy, or, frequently, a possible brain tumor. Or physicians label them with the varied tags of hysteria, anxiety neurosis, or "just nerves." Every diagnosis I have listed was once pinned on one of my friends. Some symptoms of multiple sclerosis can be confused with other illnesses, real or imagined. Multiple sclerosis, for instance, often is accompanied by extreme fatigue and strange sensations, but so is hysteria. Dr. John F. Kurtzke, who is chief of the neurology service at the Veterans Administration Hospital in Washington, D.C., and professor of neurology at Georgetown University School of Medicine, remarked that hysteria has been labeled multiple sclerosis and vice versa by even the most sophisticated observers.

Patients often fail to connect one ailment with another, to sense the significance of the pattern. A girl may see black spots like cockroaches scrambling up the wall but nothing else happens for years until she sees the top of the lamp shade but not the base.

"All of us doctors," said Dr. Kurtzke, "have had patients who suddenly recalled, after numerous medical histories had been taken, the few weeks of double vision or other symptoms they had ten, twenty, or even thirty years before what had been taken as the onset of multiple sclerosis."

The psychologist Dr. Uhlmann rationalized his own difficulties for ten years before he asked for help. It took two more years to reach a diagnosis. "I honestly felt nothing was wrong. The incidents always seemed to occur after I had been skiing or studying hard. My headaches and double vision I'd attribute to reading late at night. My leg cramps, I told myself, came from skiing. I'd fabricate reasons for my falls, my dragging foot, even bladder problems. When I lost vision in my left eye, the ophthalmologist told me to put a patch over my eye and see a neurologist, so I went through all the neurological tests, and when it was over, I knew as little as when I went in. Six months later when the patch came off my eye, my vision was restored. It wasn't until two years later, when I was associated with a neurologist, that I mentioned my leg and eye problems and he asked to examine me. After giving me a spinal tap and studying my medical records, he called me in, and I'll never forget his words. 'I have labeled your illness multiple sclerosis. Your limbs are affected, but your profession is largely vocal. You won't be able to do some things, but you are going to get more out of life than you think. I don't think you'll be snowed.' "

John Kramer—tall, straight, with the voice and bearing of a man people instinctively want to salute—was East Coast manager for one of the giants of the electronics industry. When Kramer and I met, he was riding his Amigo, a sort of scooter designed by the husband of a victim of multiple sclerosis in Michigan. He embarked on the story of a woman who stopped him as he was tootling around a shopping center on his Amigo. " 'Young man,' she said to me, 'you should be ashamed of yourself, riding around on a child's toy!' I told her, 'Madame, you have made me the happiest man in the world.' " And his laughter boomed through my apartment because the woman never realized he could not walk.

Kramer found out about multiple sclerosis when he was forty-eight years old, but he guesses he must have had it since his twenties. "Heat was an early problem with me. I had this excessive perspiration. Then, as time progressed, what I thought was just clumsiness came more often. I'd kick my left ankle bone with my right heel. My right leg was worse than my left, so three or four times a month I'd have a bloody left ankle bone—bloody literally." I laughed with him because for a long while, I, too, had a bloody left ankle bone. Kramer gave me another clue to share. "When I'd go down a long flight of steps," he said, "I'd amuse myself by tapping my foot on each step. I'd go *clickety, clickety, click* down the steps and all of a sudden I couldn't do that anymore."

That sounded familiar. "I wondered why I couldn't tap dance anymore," I told him. "I can't do the Charleston either."

Kramer nodded. "It's a matter of coordination," he said. "I suddenly lost the coordination to tap. That bothered me, but I stacked it up to old age. By then, I was in my mid forties. The first sign that sent me to a doctor didn't come for a few more years."

He and his wife, Elizabeth, were bicyclists, working up to a hundred miles in eight hours or a day. They were at fifty-five miles every weekend when multiple sclerosis hit him on one of his frequent business trips to Europe. On a Sunday morning, in Copenhagen, he was walking to a church when his legs gave out. "Here we'd cycled over fifty miles the previous weekend and now two blocks were too much for me!" Back in the States, a doctor advised vitamins. Then Kramer was off again, this time to Saudi Arabia. He remembers lying in a bathtub one day, controlling the water faucets with his feet. "When I stuck my foot under the running water to see whether it was hot or cold, I couldn't tell. I had to sit up and put my hand under the faucet to test the temperature because my foot didn't feel anything." Kramer went on to Teheran, but by then he was getting terribly fatigued just climbing stairs. He could no longer control his bladder. "My doctor told me the bladder was the big key, and this time a neurosurgeon put me in the hospital for a spinal tap."

Kramer's usually amiable face turned grim. "He's one of the top neurosurgeons in the Washington area," he said, "but he's a clod when it comes to a bedside manner. Elizabeth saw him first and asked him how I was. He told her I had a progressive neurological disease. Then he stepped on the elevator, leaving her standing there in shock." More about doctors later.

Fortunately for Kramer, his wife's grandfather was dean of a medical school. He got them swiftly to a recently retired neurologist with the time and the wisdom to tell them what they needed to know. In the four hours they spent with him, he examined Kramer to determine that he had multiple sclerosis, then explained that the disease could either progress or follow an exacerbating-remitting course. He freed them from unpleasant surprises.

Were I to try to list every possible symptom, all healthy persons would recognize a symptom as their own and cry, "Why, I have multiple sclerosis!" They don't, but it is because some signs of the disease also signal other disorders that doctors spend so long ruling out everything else their patients may have. Even when they fix on that diagnosis, they may reverse themselves later, or another physician may second-guess them. Sometimes doctors will say, as they have said to me, "If I had known you had scotoma [what I called my jigsaw-puzzle vision], I could have told you it was multiple sclerosis." Or, as they have told some of my friends who have the disease, "The bladder was the tip-off."

Of course, they are diagnosing after the fact; symptoms by themselves are usually not enough to produce a diagnosis of multiple sclerosis—particularly if they are the kind only the patient knows. Physicians want evidence they can verify by neurological tests before they are ready to put a name to what caused the patient such discomfort or embarrassment or help-lessness. So intent do some get on their process of elimination, they may say—as they bluntly told mother's friend Lois— "You've either got multiple sclerosis or a brain tumor." Some tumors are said to be notorious for causing symptoms so similar to multiple sclerosis they sometimes even follow the same pattern of appearing and disappearing. At a rap session of persons with multiple sclerosis where several complained that their physicians had frightened them by talk of brain tumors, the husband of one woman contended that doctors mention a possibly fatal illness as the alternative diagnosis just to make patients with multiple sclerosis feel relieved when they are told they are not terminally ill. A nurse, who happens to be a fellow patient, shouted, "Not true!"

The period of waiting for their physician to solve the mystery of their symptoms can be the worst time. Bewildered by unfamiliar sensations, they feel more alone than they have ever been or possibly will ever be again. If they say their legs feel encased in cement or ask for a heating pad to wrap around an arm freezing cold in the summer heat, family and friends eye them strangely. So they keep quiet.

Here are the primary symptoms in head-to-toe order—not as the physician sees them but as patients feel them:

Brain: Physicians try to determine where the protective coating of myelin has sloughed off the nerve fiber, but for the patient it is enough to know that if they laugh at a sad story and cry over a comedy it may be an MS reaction. One of my friends is called "Giggles" in her office because almost anything can set her off. I find myself crying over a military march. Others, men and women, say their feelings are hurt much more easily than they used to be. One of the men told me he can take the big changes in his life but if his wife leaves the top off the toothpaste or her stockings hanging on the bath

rod, he is ready to climb walls. Frequently, people with multiple
sclerosis start a sentence and forget, halfway through, what they were
going to say. That happens to me, too, although I wonder how much
of that is simply a sign of advancing years. I will drop a letter in the
mail slot down the hall and, only minutes later, look around for the
letter to mail. Or checks will be returned because I forgot to sign
them. Multiple sclerosis or middle age? Robert D. Douglas, former
virologist at the National Institutes of Health, told me that he trans-
poses numbers. That was the way I found out why the telephone recording so often tells me, "The number you called is out of service.
Please dial again." Like Douglas, I was transposing numbers.

Most people have heard about euphoria at one end of the emotional
spectrum and depression at the other. Those mental illnesses, according
to several specialists, rarely apply to people with multiple sclerosis.
Dr. Kurtzke says that what these persons do have in many cases is
eutonia. "The patient appears to accept his illness better than we think
we would if we were afflicted by it."

Eyes: One of the most frequent first signs of multiple sclerosis is
a change in the optic nerve. Donna Matzureff saw flashes of light
shooting from the corners of her eyes. Another girl kept brushing at
what she thought was a hair in her eye. It was the first indication she
was going blind. For many, eye troubles are fleeting. Sometimes they
come and go, sometimes they come and stay. One brief phenomenon
is the blurred vision that may follow a hot bath. Sometimes the eyes
play different tricks years apart. My jigsaw-puzzle vision, or scotoma,
came and went fifteen years before the attack of double vision, or
diplopia. (Medical terms are used occasionally to help recognize what
the doctor *means.*) Alma Gaghan lost sight in one eye and recovered
it, but the other eye went blind and never recovered. When another
girl's depth perception went, the only way she could tell whether the
coffee cup was full was by putting her finger in it. A number lose their
peripheral vision and can see only what is directly in front of them. A
fairly frequent symptom is nystagmus—eyeballs that roll around in a
way the patient notices but cannot control.

Ears: Sometimes hearing is partially lost, but, more frequently,
the reason patients are sent to ear specialists is because they start
complaining of dizziness or vertigo. As Tony Rodolakis and I both
discovered, ear specialists may diagnose a patient's dizziness as middle-
ear infection or Ménière's disease when the trouble is multiple sclerosis.

Occasionally, hearing is not less but so much more acute that any sound brings pain. A redheaded girl from Scotland in my yoga class had to give up a front-row seat at a fashion show because even the muted sound of background music was too painful.

Speech: Multiple sclerosis can make people slur their words occasionally like drunks. Sometimes a voice becomes high and nasal. Or stuttering may start or words come out garbled. A friend's speech moved from nasal to garbled, but with patience and her husband's help she still makes herself understood. In severe cases, speech may be lost entirely. Rita Dalton can no longer talk or move her hands to write, but she has been able to communicate over the years with her four children by winking and blinking her eyes.

Mouth: The tongue gives some the impression it has twisted around. Numbness may strike the upper lip. Some lose their sense of taste and some have difficulty swallowing.

Arms: Uncontrollable tremors may shake the arms. Because coordination may be lacking, hands may knock over things they reach for. As noted, a prickling sensation can run up and down the arms, or they may become scorchingly hot or freezing cold or lose all feeling for a while. Numbness in the fingers may be fleeting but come often enough to create a china cabinet full of mismatched dishes and chipped cups. Buttoning buttons, tieing shoelaces, threading needles, may become lost arts—at least temporarily. Help may be needed to cut meat or comb hair.

Bladder: Even the less affected may have an urgent need to make frequent trips to the bathroom. Bladder problems range from being unable to go to a frequent, unpredictable need. One girl said she suddenly needed a bathroom while she was standing in a long grocery check-out line. Finally, when she could control herself no longer, she noticed a small girl eyeing her with an unmistakable message on her face: "You, too?" A man used his handicap to advantage when he spent the night on a surveillance assignment with narcotics agents staked out in a van. They wanted to know why he seemed so comfortable when they had become miserably aware of the call of nature. He explained that because of multiple sclerosis, he used a bladder bag with his penis as the faucet. They seemed so interested that he wondered how they were going to put bladder bags on their expense accounts.

Bowel: Multiple sclerosis can bring on constipation or, occasionally, just the opposite. Fortunately, physicians now can deal with both conditions.

Impotence: Sexual desire remains, but whether for physical or psychological reasons, sexual performance may decrease. Like other symptoms, this varies from person to person, but may show itself by inability to achieve or sustain an erection or reach orgasm. Since most men I know with multiple sclerosis are fathers, impotence obviously did not affect them. Among females, frigidity is rarely a problem. (See chapter 4, "Love, Sex, Marriage, and Children.")

Legs: Stiffened legs are among the most common signs of multiple sclerosis; they get worse with inactivity. Even an eight-hour sleep leaves the legs stiffer on arising, one reason why having to get up during the night to go to the bathroom is not all bad. Many learn to stand for a few seconds to get their balance until their legs limber up. Leg jerks and involuntary spasms bother some people, particularly after they have been lying down. Legs may feel weak or burning or so cold that even water scalding enough to blister fails to warm them. Some complain of "bands around the knee." Some legs become so cramped that it takes a strong person to straighten them out.

Feet: Frequently a foot drops, causing a shuffle or dragging of a foot, sometimes leading to stumbling and falling. When a person with the disease sits on the floor and tries to line up her toes, she notices that one foot may droop no matter how much she struggles to keep it from flopping. She may prefer to walk in the street to avoid curbs that seem too high to clear. Some lose all sensation in their feet, as John Kramer did.

Fatigue: Of all the persons I have met, not one has escaped the fatigue that drains in a way no person without the disease can visualize. Gerry Shur of the Justice Department likened his fatigue to all the water suddenly being drained out of the bathtub. Elaine Dewar talked about a fatigue so encompassing she would spend eighteen hours a day sleeping.

Pain: The only pain I ever had from multiple sclerosis was from bones broken in falls, and not many I met talked about pain either. Some, however, suffer from severe headaches, backaches, or arm and leg cramps. Radiating pains down the spine and into the legs occur at times. Patients may try acupuncture, usually with meager success. What happens more often is typical—the pain may simply disappear, at least for a time.

What triggers or precipitates an attack? Many, perhaps prodded by an interested physician, believe they can trace an attack of multiple sclerosis to some crisis or a time of stress. It could be the emotional shock of sudden death, too much work crammed into too little time, the loss of a needed job, a big night on the town, a hot day on the beach, or a fever-producing infection.

Two leading German neurologists, after studying more than twelve hundred patients, reported that more than 60 percent experienced their first symptoms during military service or in a particular stress situation in Germany during World War II. Many had their first bout or an exacerbation of multiple sclerosis during a dangerous or strenuous military operation, a bombardment, a disorganized retreat, or other anxious time.

Physicians and researchers hesitate to make any flat statement about what may trigger an attack. Dr. Henry McFarland, a National Institutes of Health neurologist, cautiously agreed—after I cited specific cases of friends—that in some individuals there seems to be a fairly clear relationship between stress and a true exacerbation, when an individual under a good deal of stress develops a new symptom. "But many multiple sclerosis patients under tremendous stress do not exacerbate. We are not talking about a clear-cut relationship."

Dr. Russell N. DeJong, chairman of the neurology department at the University of Michigan Medical School and former chairman of the National Multiple Sclerosis Society's medical advisory board, came closer to the experiences of persons I know when he said emotional upsets seem to bring on flare-ups.

Sometimes, there is no permanent harm; other times, an attack can be disastrous. Robert S. Clark knows what emotional

shock can do. He was so handy with the tools of many trades
that he had five licenses and became building manager of a
Montgomery County, Maryland, high school—the first black
to hold the job—when illness forced his early retirement. He
had escaped from his wheelchair for the third time and was
talking about working again when he lost the father who had
been the model for his life. That put him back in his wheelchair. You will meet him again, because he is not licked yet.

Jeane Hofheimer, once women's golf champion of her club,
was using a wheelchair only for distances when her father died
suddenly. "My left leg had been pretty good," she said. "I could
use it to drag my right leg, and all of a sudden, after dad's
death, my left leg just stopped. I used to be able to get in and
out of the wheelchair myself, stand up in the shower, sit on the
clothes hamper to wash my face. After the funeral, I couldn't
do any of those things." The doctor ordered an eight-hour nurse.
"Outside of that, my doctor says I'm the healthiest person he
knows." Jeane is simply too busy to feel sorry for herself, with
her golf tournaments for the benefit of multiple sclerosis research and the thousands of sweaters she has managed to get
knitted for needy children. To keep some golf in her own life,
she has learned to putt from a wheelchair with her left hand.
Jeane, too, will reappear later.

Emotional stress does not always stem from sorrow. Dr.
Kathleen Shanahan Cohen had barely weathered the trauma of
fire sweeping her family's summer home when she was named
New Jersey's Medical Woman of the Year. She attributes the
overwhelming fatigue that followed to a "tremendous emotional high." Her psychiatric training prompted her to speculate that an excess even of joy might prove costly to a person
with multiple sclerosis.

What about automobile accidents? When I told Dr. Kurtzke
that a number of friends with multiple sclerosis seemed to get
their first attack after an automobile accident, he cautioned

against jumping to cause-and-effect conclusions. Dr. McFarland of NIH agreed. "We have to guard against an individual's tendency to relate the onset of the disease to something he clearly remembers during that period. If the first symptom occurred after an accident, it's easy to relate the two, but unless somebody could go through all the cases of MS and say how many actually started after a traumatic episode, it's very difficult to assign cause and effect."

Anne Jackson made the cause-and-effect connection long before any doctor said she had multiple sclerosis. Anne, black and brilliant (IQ 165), was studying to become a mortician when a classroom door toppled over, striking her in the head. Before the accident, she had occasionally felt a tingling sensation in her hands and legs but a complete physical examination had found nothing wrong. After the accident, she lost control of bladder and bowel and all sensation in her arms. When she left the hospital three weeks later, she could not stand light in her eyes, could not balance herself. "I felt like I was dragging concrete blocks on either side of my body," Anne said. "I would burn myself or cut myself and not even know it." She had herself admitted to another hospital and insisted on all the tests related to neurological problems. A neurologist gave her the diagnosis.

Some experiences can accentuate whatever is already wrong, make weakened legs weaker, vision more blurred, fatigue more draining. Physicians may tell their patients to stay away from people with colds, try to avoid emotional upsets or exhaustion, but, as I learned from scary experience, they do not always mention extremes of heat and cold such as saunas and ice-cold movie houses. It was a sauna that got me. Perhaps this sauna was hotter than usual or I stayed in it longer or my reactions had changed. When I crawled out of the wooden bed and tried to stand, my legs folded under me. The manager of the spa brought in a nurse. "No more saunas for you," she said. "You have high blood pressure." By the time I visited my own doctor, my blood pressure was normal, and so were my legs.

I discovered saunas were out along with sunbathing and very hot baths. My stockbroker friend Tony Rodolakis told me that summer heat would make him "delirious" with fatigue.

"I'd climb on a bus after work, push my way to the stairwell and sit on the step because this bus was always too crowded for me to find a seat and I couldn't stand. At my apartment building, I'd look down my corridor to make sure no one was coming and I'd get down and crawl to my door. I'd fall in my apartment and lie there maybe half an hour, too exhausted even to unfasten my jacket.

"When I finally managed to reach my bed and started to unbutton my shirt, I was so exhausted I couldn't unbutton more than one button without resting a minute or two. I'd feel hungry but when I finally put something in the oven, I'd have to lie down and rest again. Knowing my food was hot, I'd tell myself if I didn't get up, it would burn and I would have wasted all that energy. I'd pour a glass of milk but feel too tired to pick up the glass. I'd turn on the television set but feel too tired to watch it. I'd tell myself I can't go through another day like this. Then, I'd wake up in the morning and say to myself, 'Hey, I feel pretty good. I think I'll go to work.' And I'd go through the same damn thing again. I look back and say, 'How did I do it? I must have been crazy.' "

Dr. McFarland explained what might be going on: "Once an individual has an attack and loses myelin [the fatty insulation around the nerve fiber], that myelin for the most part never completely regenerates, so the patient is left with a small area of abnormal nerve fibers and there's some difficulty with transmitting messages to that area. When the patient starts to recover, probably there's some rerouting of information and conduction of messages goes back to a somewhat more normal situation. There seem to be some situations, however, which make it more difficult for messages to go through, and one of these is temperature change. So when we talk about patients becoming weaker in hot weather, it doesn't always represent a true exacerbation. It's not a new attack of the disease but probably an accentuation of disease already there."

On a summer Sunday, Dorothy Cox visited the local movie house in her short cotton dress. She could feel the air conditioner blowing cold air across her legs. The next night at work in the library, there was a sharp cramp in her left thigh. "The pain was so excruciating I had to go home. I couldn't get in or out of bed, couldn't turn. My doctor prescribed aspirin and a muscle relaxant, which did absolutely no good. I was in such agony I couldn't work." She began physical therapy three times a week and, finally, the inner thigh, where the trouble had started, relaxed, but she never felt able to go back to work.

Lucy Handler, whose husband, Dr. Philip Handler, is now president of the National Academy of Sciences, discovered what an evening of square dancing can do while she was a faculty wife at Duke University. "We had danced until two A.M. the night before I was to introduce Mrs. Franklin D. Roosevelt at a meeting. She had made her speech and I had thanked her and asked for questions from the floor when, suddenly, I had to hang on to the rostrum. The young mayor of Durham, North Carolina, was on the platform with me, so I whispered, 'Please help me. If I let go of this stand, I'll fall.' He took the questions and closed the meeting, standing there with me hanging on his arm. He drove me right to Duke Hospital." At that point, although Lucy Handler's husband knew and the doctors at the hospital knew she had multiple sclerosis, she was not told. "My husband says I did not want to know, because I certainly had enough knowledge by then to know if I wanted to."

Timothy Drury, now a prosecutor in Buffalo, was nineteen and going into his junior year at Georgetown University when he spent the summer as a garbage man. He noticed the fatigue in his legs, but ignored it and began his junior year. The weakness in his legs continued. Now he had insomnia and other bothersome problems as well. "Doctors at the Georgetown clinic told me it was just nerves, so during the Christmas break I worked as a mailman, walking a lot, and all the fatigue came back to my legs." Back home in Buffalo, two doctors assured him nothing was wrong; a third told him he had a slipped disc but that there was one chance in a hundred it might be multiple sclerosis. It was.

Infections, a constant threat, can precipitate a full-blown attack. I had a small taste of the effect of something foreign in the system after my swine-flu shot. The next day, when the room swam around me and the dizziness made me afraid to move, I thought, *Could this be the exacerbation they tell me about?* I called my doctor's nurse to ask. "Oh, you shouldn't believe everything you read," she said, obviously referring to newspaper accounts of swine-flu deaths. "You don't understand," I moaned, "I *want* the dizziness to come from the swine-flu vaccine." She assured me the vaccine could indeed make me dizzy and it was nothing to worry about. After that reassurance, the dizziness disappeared.

Brenetta Payne was fired after six and a half years on the job, and soon afterwards, presumably from the shock of being fired, she found that her legs wouldn't hold her up. "I wound up in the hospital." Because Brenetta never ends a conversation on a downer, she hastened to add, "The happiest thing that ever happened to me was seeing my toes wriggling again."

Jewell Philips, whom Brenetta was to befriend, had no idea
why she felt the way she did, but she knows how it began.
The firm she was working for had lost its government contract and her job was "driving me crazy." By the time she
was admitted to a hospital, the muscles in her face had "relaxed or something, because my face had fallen down to the
side. One of my eyes was on top of my head and the other
was frozen in one position. I was paralyzed down my left
side, had no taste in my mouth, and thought I was dying."
She was put on the psychiatric ward because "everybody
thought I was just having a nervous breakdown," but after
a number of tests, her family was told she had multiple
sclerosis.

"I was so grateful to have something that somebody else
had. Until then, I had never heard of multiple sclerosis, but
just telling me I had a known disease made me feel good."

Symptoms may last only as long as the stress persists, as
my dizziness had. One girl I know dreaded her mother's
upcoming visit because she did not want her mother to try
to do everything for her. When her mother arrived, the girl's
walk became a lurch and she could barely lift her legs to
climb stairs. As soon as her mother left, her gait improved.
Stairs were no longer a problem. Her problem was not the
myelin disappearing, as in a genuine attack, but mama appearing.

The stresses of everyday life may have an exaggerated impact. Yet many victims keep going where lesser ones would
falter. Nancy Lewis was a technician at the Library of Congress and the train she took to work was a third of a mile
from the nearest taxi. Although she had two canes, by the
time she reached her office she was exhausted. Despite a
baby at home she needed her job. "I know I'm not getting
enough rest," Nancy admitted. "I'm not sure whether it's
the way I manage my life or the progress of the disease, but

since the baby came and I went back to work I'm getting
slowly but progressively worse." You will meet Nancy again
to find out how she solved her problem.

The course of multiple sclerosis varies as much as the
symptoms and what triggers them. For some, the disease
follows a gradually progressive course. As one husband said
of his wife, "It's been a slowly downhill thing. She'd hold
on to my arm, then a cane, then I'd come home to find her
crawling on the floor. She used a wheelchair in the beginning
only when she went out. Now she uses it inside and out."
For a minority, the downhill course is sharp and unremitting.
On the other hand, some people I know who had a bad time,
bedeviled by several symptoms, now have been free of the
disease for years.

Just as no foolproof method yet exists for diagnosis, no one
can be certain of the course and outcome. Some doctors,
however, now believe that the pattern established during the
first three to five years of the disease reflects its future course.
Dr. Kurtzke and his colleagues now are trying to document
that course. Their study covers 572 World War II veterans
who had been diagnosed as having multiple sclerosis in service.
In surveying these veterans fifteen years after onset, Dr.
Kurtzke found that among those severely disabled five years
after onset, nearly all were still severely disabled ten and
fifteen years later. Among those moderately disabled, fewer
than half had progressed to severe disablement. And of those
with little or no disability at five years, only one in ten had
become severely disabled. Dr. Kurtzke now hopes to find out
whether the score at fifteen years after onset still holds at
thirty years. What he is measuring is the severity of the disease, not how the person got there, whether by progressive or
recurrent course. "Being able to predict the outcome of MS,"
he said, "can have a very positive therapeutic effect on the
patient."

Dr. Kurtzke knows his patients and how much they yearn for certainty. If a doctor can use scientific criteria proven over a thirty-year test to predict the outcome of the disease, he may be able to give patients the reassurance now so lacking. That, too, could be a marker on the road to hope, for uncertainty can breed perplexity, even despair. Dr. Kurtzke was the first expert on multiple sclerosis I met whose entire attitude radiated hope.

Research such as Dr. Kurtzke's is a comforting antidote to medical myth and to popular misconceptions like those in three publications I heard about. An army wife with multiple sclerosis had read an article in the *Army Times* about military insurance. It showed a patient in a wheelchair, and in the second paragraph, it said the disease is eventually fatal. "To print something like that is so discouraging to MS patients who might read it, so detrimental." From the catch in her voice, I knew it was at least detrimental to her.

And in, of all places, a health magazine, an article reviewing a new diet book for victims of multiple sclerosis said flatly: "The outlook is often hopelessly bleak; an abbreviated life span of progressive muscular and sensory deterioration spent largely in a wheelchair . . . within 10 or 12 years after the onset of the disease, the patient usually loses the ability to walk."

One girl I know had gone to the only medical dictionary she could find, a 1959 edition, when her neurologist seemed to be evading her questions. She found this definition: "A progressive disabling disease of the central nervous system, characterized by temporary remissions, gradual intensification of symptoms and eventual paralysis." More recent medical dictionaries do not make such all-inclusive statements about multiple sclerosis, but the older volumes are still on library shelves.

When he was put in the hospital, my friend Gerry Shur

was convinced he was going to die. A West Virginia woman told me she wrote a last letter to her children from her hospital bed. Both are fully alive today.

Some physicians, particularly those long out of medical school, still subscribe to the discredited killer myth. When they took their medical training, people were dying of the effects of multiple sclerosis. Sylvia Lawry, then twenty-one, first ran into that myth when she took her young brother, Bernard, to one of New York's most eminent neurosurgeons to find out what caused his succession of strange ailments. The doctor said the boy had a rare disease known as multiple sclerosis, that he'd be lucky to live five more years, and there was nothing he could do about it. The year was 1936. At that time people didn't survive long with multiple sclerosis. A 1936 report shows that for 30 percent of patients life expectancy was then only two to four years. Only 8 percent lived more than twenty years, and only 4 percent more than thirty years.

Sylvia Lawry has devoted her life to changing those statistics. Her brother lived for thirty-seven years after that death sentence was passed. She founded and remains executive director of the National Multiple Sclerosis Society. Research spurred by the society has definitely disproved that the disease itself is a killer.

Most medical authorities now agree. Infections that used to kill are now prevented or treated before they get out of hand. Active physiotherapy and exercise keep patients functioning; medical and social care have vastly improved; and as one international authority put it, "The MS patient is learning to abandon his role of the passive sufferer and is taking an active part in providing help for himself and fellow victims."

The National Institute of Neurological and Communicative Disorders and Stroke (NINCDS), the government agency

that the National Multiple Sclerosis Society played a major
role in founding, should be the last word. "MS is not a
killer," said their recent pamphlet on multiple sclerosis. "In
fact, the majority of persons with MS can expect to live their
normal life span."

We now know also that the disease does not always
paralyze, does not always progress. Autopsies of some men
who died from other causes in late middle age showed a
classic picture of nerve coverings damaged by multiple sclerosis in men who never even knew they had the disease.

Recent studies, cited in the NINCDS pamphlet,* indicate
that at least half of those with multiple sclerosis, fifteen to
twenty years after the onset of the disease, can still do most
of what they did before onset. Of the other half, some have
a slowly progressive disease. Only a small percentage develops
a more rapid, severely incapacitating form of multiple sclerosis.

Mayo Clinic studies reported that 74 percent of a group
studied there were still able to walk around twenty years
after their first attack. From all the new studies, Dr. Joe R.
Brown of Mayo Clinic's section of neurology has concluded
that multiple sclerosis is considerably less devastating on the
average than had been believed. His pamphlet, "Who Says
Multiple Sclerosis Patients Can't Work?," is as sunny in its
point of view as its bright yellow cover.

Nor are the fears of insanity justified. Only in rare cases is
the brain itself affected. Although one encyclopedia recently
speculated that victims seem optimistic possibly because of
the effect of the disease on the brain—it gave no credit to
hope or courage!—Dr. Wallace W. Tourtellotte, an authority
on multiple sclerosis who heads the neurology service at a
California VA hospital, counters such distortions. "Fortu-

* *Multiple sclerosis, hope through research;* National Institute of Neurological and Communicative Disorders and Stroke, Bethesda, Md. 20014.

nately," he said, "multiple sclerosis rarely affects the patient's memory or ability to think logically."

Victims of multiple sclerosis can overcome fear and arrive at serenity, acceptance, and hope. Mrs. John Kramer, who has weathered her husband's disease, says that diagnosis itself is a relief. "We could never get the house cold enough for him. We'd be wearing heavy sweaters and he was perspiring. Now he's like everybody else." She believes patients go through a series of stages in adjusting to the disease. The first stage is withdrawal—"an attempt to escape from everything around you." Next comes an extreme reaction, "as the full impact hits." Then comes a desire to reverse one's lifestyle. Then comes the question, "Why me? Why did this have to happen to me?" Then comes a search for every possible alternative treatment. Then husband and wife struggle to express what is happening to them.

"Then, all of a sudden, you think, *Oh, the hell with it,* and you settle down into it like a rocking chair and it's part of you like having one blue eye and one brown eye, and you live with it and you don't make such a big deal of it. The anticipation of the inevitable sometimes can be worse than the reality. The game of pretense is over."

As a nurse, Pauline Schultz knew tomorrow could be better or worse than today, but still she found it hard to believe in the miracle of remission. After six years of multiple sclerosis, the miracle happened last spring. "We noticed the difference in my ability to do things, and last summer, I was able to hike a mile with the children up a mountain stream. It's hard to describe how you feel because it's an inward feeling of wanting to burst. You feel like a rose, a beautiful rosebud. And now that I am feeling better I'm opening up to enjoy the full life. It's wonderful to hike in the woods, take off my shoes and walk up the middle of a cold stream."

Chapter 3

Family, Friends, and Enemies

In the candle glow of an empty church, a father made his daughter's dearest wish a reality. He knew she needed a wheelchair, but he gave her the confidence to walk down the aisle on her wedding day like any other bride.

And he was the man who could do it; he had coached winning teams for years at Notre Dame. Now Ara Parseghian and his daughter, Karen, were the team, and he approached this challenge like any other game. First, there was the fight talk, low-keyed but effective. Karen did not believe she could make it to the altar rail. Her father suggested mildly that his players drew confidence from seeing what they could accomplish in practice. Why didn't they just try it—just the two of them—when no one was around to make her self-conscious or see her falter. But of course she wouldn't falter, not her father's daughter.

That slow march to the altar rail was the longest twenty yards of Ara Parseghian's coaching career and the most radiantly successful. The next day, Karen made it down the aisle on her father's arm.

Multiple sclerosis has struck Parseghian's family three times —his sister and a brother-in-law before his daughter—and he has been fighting back for years. He has served on the national board of the National Multiple Sclerosis Society, as national campaign chairman and national sports committee chairman. He has headed the "Athletes *vs.* MS" program and made the sports world intensely aware that what happens to so many young people could happen to any of them. As a consequence every season produces a new crop of sports stars who raise funds for research.

His total commitment is what Sylvia Lawry, the founder and executive director of the National Multiple Sclerosis Society, has visualized for all families hit with multiple sclerosis. She expects them to react as she did when her brother was stricken, to make a lasting commitment to finding the cause and cure. And many of them have. From the beginning of the society over three decades ago, thousands of relatives of the stricken ones have given their name, money, and energy to finance research and to help victims live as fully as they can. So far, they cannot buy a cure but they can buy hope— and that is what Sylvia Lawry offers.

She realized that important people mean important contributions as well as access to other important people, and, in the name of multiple sclerosis research, she found them. She has used all the influence she could muster through these family connections not only for fund-raising but to stimulate government interest in more research directed specifically at multiple sclerosis. Somewhere among these families one can trace the impetus behind establishment of the congressionally mandated National Advisory Commission on Multiple Sclerosis and the National Institute of Neurological and Communicative Disorders and Stroke.

A number of notables, from bank presidents to movie stars, get involved because the disease seems more often to strike at the rich, the well-educated, and the talented. So Shirley Temple Black, child star turned ambassador, became national and international chairman of volunteers after her brother was stricken; and Ray A. Kroc, founder and chairman of the board of McDonald's, pledged a million dollars in his continuing search for cause and cure since his sister was stricken. And Daniel J. Haughton, chairman of the board of Lockheed Aircraft, served as chairman of the board of the National Multiple Sclerosis Society, its president, and chairman of its multimillion-dollar research development fund because his wife has multiple sclerosis. And guest pianist Bertica Shulman Cramer, performing with Boston Pops conductor Arthur Fiedler at "MS Night at the Pops," dedicated the concert to her husband, a multiple sclerosis patient.

The list of rich and talented is more than matched by the less wealthy and talented but equally concerned relatives who promote fashion shows, concerts, walkathons, dance marathons, and the hugely successful MS READ-a-thon in their hometowns. The *MS Messenger*, newsletter of the National Multiple Sclerosis Society, periodically salutes their achievements in a column, "All in the MS Family."

If there is to be any hope for its victims, multiple sclerosis must be a family affair. Parseghian knows it; so does the mother who gets her club to make a thousand hard-candy wreaths to sell at Christmastime so the Multiple Sclerosis Society can buy wheelchairs. So does the small son of a patient who gets his neighbors to pledge a contribution for each book he reads in the READ-a-thon. There are, however, others with multiple sclerosis in the family who refuse to admit it even to themselves, or go to the other extreme and overprotect their daughters, sisters, or husbands into wheelchairs and back rooms. Instead of encouraging them to work to their limit, these relatives try to narrow their limits, make invalids out of people who are really quite well except for some times when they are sick.

Many who confided in me were so resentful of the way their families dealt with their disorder that I leave them nameless except for one woman who has gone through the travail of denying the disease, ranting against it, crying "Why me?," trying to bargain with God, plunging into depression, finally accepting and reaching now for hope.

"My husband and I went through the stages together," said Lori Sanjiau, who works for Social Security but composes songs and plays the flute to her husband's guitar accompaniment. "My mother is still denying." Lori believes that families go through the same phases as victims but that it is harder on the family. "*I'm* going to live with it, but they see it happening. I feel luckier than they because I know I can cope with it. I wind up comforting my family and friends. . . . I think it's a lot easier to live with MS as a patient than as a parent.

"Facing MS is a grieving process, a way of coping with a loss." Her family is growing to accept her disease. "As a family we have found a great deal of inner strength. We pass it around and it seems to help everyone. It's a slow, gradual process. For us, the change began one night when I was crying wildly and screaming, 'Why me, why did this happen to me? It's not fair.' After I got it out of my system, and my husband got the same fears out of his system, we felt calm. We could say it's okay."

Lori's recipe for dealing with the disease as a family: "Talk it out."

If it's all out in the open, that it's nobody's fault and nobody's to blame, Lori reasons, then people with MS will get over the feeling that the disease was foisted on them because there's something bad about them.

When I asked Alma Gaghan, a mother of seven, how she thought family and friends could be most helpful, she also replied, "By talking about it. Plain and simple. Not catering to me or giving me more affection than ordinarily they gave me, but talking about it."

If parents talk about the disease at all, and many prefer

not to, they will frequently say they find it difficult to deal with a disease of unknown cause, unpredictable course, and limited treatment. They could adjust to a disease with specific symptoms, but with this one, they do not know how to act. So they keep saying to the doctors, "Are you certain?" or they go on doctor-shopping, cure-hunting expeditions. They overwhelm their stricken relatives with care before they need it, undermine their self-esteem, leaving behind resentment rather than reassurance.

As time passes, both family and patients may get confused about their roles. The family sees a girl looking as well as ever without realizing how weak and fatigued she really is and they feel fortified in their denial that anything is wrong. The patient, feeling fine one day but hurting and miserable the next, is alternately resentful of oversolicitous relatives when she feels perfectly able to do for herself or bitterly hurt when no one offers help when she needs it most.

A neurologist of note says the way the family and others respond may have a greater impact on the patient's psychological attitudes and behavior than the patient's own feelings. Parents who refuse to accept that anything is really wrong with their son or daughter can literally make them sick.

The mother-in-law of one of my MS friends accused her of cheating her husband by marrying him, and when the girl told her father-in-law that his son had beaten her, the man said she probably deserved it. More typical, however, is the mother-in-law who took a second job so she could keep up payments on her son's house when he lost his job and she could see that his wife, who had multiple sclerosis, was going downhill from worry. In this most contradictory of diseases, in-laws often are more kind, considerate, and helpful than a person's own family.

One mother salves her conscience by sending her daughter money, but never invites her to visit her because she finds it depressing. Another mother obviously could not make up her mind how to behave. "She's either too sympathetic or she's giving me the devil because the house isn't cleaner, and she's after my husband to get somebody in." What hurt my friend most, though, was her mother's advising her to "be realistic" and to look for a ranch-style home because in the future she would be in a wheelchair. Since she does not even use a cane and shows no signs of needing one, her mother was the one who was not being realistic—only a puller-down.

Probably the most destructive families of all are those who try to deny the disease.

Dr. Uhlmann, who is both psychologist and patient, emphasized the damaging effects of a parent's denial. A girl he was asked to help had accepted her illness but her parents had not. The father, robust and sports-minded, thought his daughter's illness was "a stigma" on his personal life. Dr. Uhlmann told the parents that the father's rejection of his daughter would certainly have a detrimental effect on her. "She would feel like a reject. It would be a self-fulfilling prophecy because she would *be* a reject."

Once when another girl was having an attack, couldn't walk, and had no way to get from bed to bath, she sent her husband off to borrow a pair of crutches her father had. Her father wanted to know why she needed them. "She can't walk and she wants to get out of bed," the husband replied. "No," her father said. "She doesn't need them." He never talks to her about the illness. "He'll start to say to people, 'I remember she used to . . .' That's the closest he'll come to the fact that I'm not what I used to be. If I lived at home, he would put a damper on any little bit of hope I had."

A man in his twenties was watching closely as a girl, once a dancer, directed a dance performance from her wheelchair while her small boy ran around trying to be useful. Finally, he asked the young mother: "You have MS?" She said she did. "Your son says 'MS' like it's just another phrase, not a terrible disease. Does he know what it is?" She nodded vigorously. "Of course, he does. He knows all about it and he's really a big help."

The young man explained why he asked so many questions. "My mother has had multiple sclerosis for twenty years," he said. "She's very disabled, but we never talked about it. My father wouldn't let us. We three children were never asked to do anything for her. Instead, my father would bring in maids, nurses, cooks, physiotherapists. I feel so guilty now, even if it wasn't my fault. My father shielded us." To shed his guilt, he offered to help the former dancer put on a show to benefit patients with multiple sclerosis.

When the disease strikes twice in the same family, the family members either fight twice as hard to overcome it, as Ara Parseghian did, or refuse twice as vehemently to accept it. Dr. Jocelyn Gill's father was like that. Dr. Gill, who conceived the scientific space experiments for the astronauts, was the daughter of a victim. She said her father never became reconciled to her mother's illness. It took him years to accept hers.

The National Multiple Sclerosis Society now offers an eight-week course, all the way from neurology to sexuality, to give families and friends a better understanding of the illness and help them care for the people with multiple sclerosis in their lives. The course gives the healthy member of the family some recognition that he has needs, too. He wants to know how to adjust his life-style to the needs of the sick partner, to plan their future. Healthy partners and parents want to air their feeling of guilt and get help with dispelling it. "How can I avoid being a nursemaid to my wife?" "How can I have some time to myself?" "How can I continue a loving relationship with my wife when she is becoming more and more demanding?" The husband who asked that complained that whenever he tried to do something for his wife, he never did it the way she wanted it. He would do the laundry, but when it came to putting the handkerchiefs in one drawer, the stockings in another, he said he had too much to do to worry about such trifles. He bundled it all in together and his wife would become so upset she had to go to bed. Others in the group could answer that one for him. His wife was not just going overboard on a neatness kick. If she knew just where everything was, she could decide what she wanted and get it for herself with a minimum of effort. But if she had to search for it, pulling out one drawer after another, her frustration would rise while her carefully hoarded energy dwindled. No wonder a topsy-turvy drawer would send her to bed!

One man I know was so immersed in his business that he went off on a buying trip when his wife was obviously on the cutting edge of an attack. She was stumbling around the house, frightening her teen-agers by pulling things down as she grasped for anything to keep from falling. Her husband had not been gone long when her doctor ordered her to get to the hospital fast. It never occurred to him to ask and she did not volunteer that she had to drive herself from the farm to the hospital. Her knees were scraped and bleeding by the time she reached the door because she had parked on the hospital lot and, unable to walk with a bag full of books and a suitcase, she had crawled on hands and knees across the gravel to the hospital door.

In the several years since that episode, her husband has apparently graduated from his own denial that anything is really wrong with his wife. He enrolled for the first jointly sponsored MS–Red Cross home-care course in his area and drove an hour each way to get to every session, sometimes through snow. Another husband, who could afford nurses to tend his wife, nevertheless went to the course to please her. It pleased her very much.

Both parents of one young man with the disease attended

every session to learn to help him when he needs help. Until now, the son has complained bitterly that his mother gets him down by wanting to do everything for him that he can still do for himself. Presumably, by attending the course she will learn where help leaves off and hindrance begins.

John and Elizabeth Kramer had been married before and were enjoying a continuing honeymoon when John Kramer was stricken. "The families of our two marriages rallied around," Elizabeth Kramer said. "Instead of abdicating, they created opportunities to do things together. What others looked at as everyday living, we made an occasion." John added his report: "They all say that with my MS, I'm easier to get along with than before. They have a more understanding father now because we have more hours to spend with each other."

Jean Urciolo finds her in-laws going out of the way to make kind gestures. Her mother-in-law calls regularly to ask if there's anything she can do, and she means it. Since Jean's arms are not strong enough to iron, her mother-in-law sends over her own maid to iron her son's shirts. She knows her son enjoys Italian food, so when she fixes an Italian dinner, she sends over what Jean calls a CARE package. "I say she doesn't have to do that, but my husband says, 'Why discourage it?' "

Jean does not feel threatened by such gestures. She never was any good at ironing shirts, even when she was healthy, and she never could cook Italian dishes as her Italian mother-in-law does. She is grateful when her husband has to go out of town and several members of his family call to ask if she needs anything. "This is real, not phony concern," she says. "It is good to know somebody cares that much."

While Rita Dalton has gone steadily downhill to her present total helplessness, her family has never made her a stranger in her own house, has always tried in some way to keep her a part of one loving family.

"She has had a great deal of influence on our sons," said Bill Dalton. "They will talk to her about schoolwork and she gives good answers. She's very good in English. When they ask her a question, she can say a word or two. She responds with her eyes mostly. You can tell what she means by the movement of her eyelids. When she has even one degree of fever she can't say anything. So we spell words out letter by letter and her eyelids tell us whether we've got the right word. We know she's hot and we want to give her a drink so we spell words out to arrive at what she wants."

One day their daughter brought over her six-month-old baby, and Dalton put the baby on Rita's stomach. Rita smiled, the baby cooed, Rita managed to make some noises, and for a moment there, she could experience the joy of being a grandmother.

Some people are sensible enough to take an offer of help at face value. Thus, when Barbara McGrath's brother asked her if there was anything he could do for her, she promptly said yes, teach my boys how to ski. When Anne Jackson's niece asked if she wanted anything, Anne said yes, rearrange my staples and spices so I can get to them easily. Now she has everything she needs within reach of her wheelchair. That, I think, is the way it should be. The wife who went to bed in despair because her lingerie was left in a jumble by her husband, for instance, could have spared herself that distress if she had asked one of the many church members who visit her to rearrange her bureau drawers the way she likes them. To her, friends from her church are like a second family and could be used that way.

One of the oddities of this strange malady is the victims' tendency to overreact. Ordinary stress for a healthy person is extraordinary stress for them. They can gain a rich feeling of satisfaction by accomplishing a task a healthy person would find routine. Their pride is a fragile thing, easily shattered, hard to rebuild. Their feelings are hurt by small slights and careless disinterest but their gratitude is enormous for small favors. It is as if the disease, in striking at the nerves, has made their emotions as taut as violin strings, quivering at a touch.

The people who seem to fare best in this setting are those surrounded not by cloying attention but by practical, down-to-earth, sensible cooperation. How can the family cooperate most effectively? Both the experts and the victims have ideas about that, and here they are:

The family should find out enough about the disease—preferably from some authoritative source like the MS–Red Cross home-care course—to understand that people with the disease have off days and good days.

Victims are often robbed of their privacy and feel the loss bitterly. Any equipment that restores it would help to restore their worth as individuals in their own eyes. They feel particularly vulnerable in the bathroom. That should be their private domain, and for some it can be if relatives will install safety rails in the bathtub and a bath chair so patients can get in and out of the tub themselves.

With minimum effort, relatives can offer intellectual privacy, too. When vision grows more limited, as it sometimes does, ordinary news and magazine print becomes illegible, but relatives can get not only talking books free from the Library of Congress but also large-print newspapers, magazines, and newsletters. Anything to avoid a steady diet of television, particularly when the program is chosen by someone else.

When people with the disease are frustrated with their inability to do what they did before, they can regress, become indecisive and dependent, or they can force their way out of it. Two of the most handicapped men I know still are the bosses in their own homes. When Dr. Joseph J. Panzarella, Jr.'s children were growing up and came to their mother for

permission to do something, she says she always told them:
"Ask your father." Despite the fact that he can move only his
head, he remains the head of his family. Robert Clark, the
Maryland school building manager, retired from work but not
from his family responsibilities. To his wife and children, he
still calls the shots. Thus, they all go to church on Sunday.
"That's a must. When you're too big to go to church, you're
too big to stay home." They obey but they also love. "They
check on me in the morning and when they come home from
school and at night before they go out to see if I need anything." Despite being tied to a wheelchair, he is still the father
his family loves and respects. And that, probably, is why
he keeps on planning, dreaming, and building—at least he
directs the building. Both men have strong wills and great
determination, but it was their families that kept them de-
cision-makers.

The bond of marriage, at least theoretically, makes a
healthy husband or wife responsible for the ill partner's well-
being. Members of the family likewise have some obligation—
whether they recognize it or not—to care for their own. Since
the person with multiple sclerosis has no such claim on friends,
whatever friends do becomes a gift of love, freely given, grate-
fully received. The fact of having friends may have even a
physical effect. As one young man confided, "The more
friends I make, the more positive things I accomplish, the
more strength wells up inside me. I don't feel as tired at
day's end."

Some friends get lost as the paths of sick and well diverge.
Sometimes friends are afraid. Victims of multiple sclerosis
often can sense fear in their friends' eyes, fear of catching
the disease.

Joanne Bell and Jean McLean dealt with this problem patiently. Both have multiple sclerosis. Both work for the same
congressional committee. Jean was first stricken as a college

freshman, but her doctor failed to tell her why she was losing her coordination and must leave school. For the next two decades she had times of exhaustion, but her next major attack did not come until twenty-three years later, and by then she had been working for many years on Capitol Hill. Her parents are gone now, and so is the doctor, so she has no way of knowing whether he shared with them the suspicion that she had multiple sclerosis—a suspicion that surfaced when the stored records of the dead physician were searched for a clue to her medical problem.

At a nearby desk in the same office, Joanne Bell asked eagerly about Jean's symptoms. "When you put your head down," Joanne wanted to know, "do you feel a shock going through your spinal cord?" "Yes, I do," Jean told her. Joanne was beginning to suspect that some of the problems that had beset her years before Jean came to work at the committee were due to multiple sclerosis, especially the six-week period years earlier when she went blind in one eye. When Joanne wound up in the hospital only a few months after Jean's attack, her suspicions were confirmed and she called from the hospital to tell her friends in the office.

Jean carefully provided brochures from the Multiple Sclerosis Society for their friends to read so they would know it was not contagious, a natural fear with the two having attacks only months apart. The National Institute of Neurological and Communicative Disorders and Stroke asked me to suggest names of victims still working, despite their handicap, who would be willing to be photographed for a pamphlet the institute was issuing about the disease. Joanne and Jean not only agreed to go public but arranged to be pictured with two of their bosses—the chairman of the House Interstate and Foreign Commerce Committee and the chairman of the Health Subcommittee, which pushed through Congress the law establishing NINCDS, the agency for research into multiple sclerosis.

The fear that multiple sclerosis is contagious nearly cost a teacher her job. She was working part-time when somebody at the school noticed a newspaper article describing multiple sclerosis as an infectious disease. The school principal was promptly petitioned to fire her on the ground she might contaminate the children. The local Multiple Sclerosis Society had to get the chief of its medical advisory board to assure the principal that the disease might be infectious, as for example, pneumonia can be caused by a viral infection—and even multiple sclerosis's infectiousness was by no means certain— but it definitely wasn't contagious, that is, capable of transmission to others.

Dr. James Q. Simmons, then director of medical programs for the National Multiple Sclerosis Society, said he's never known a husband or wife to get the disease from a stricken mate or a doctor or nurse to catch the disease from their patients. Brothers, sisters, or other close relatives have on rare occasions been stricken—usually years apart—but researchers studying twins and other family clusters believe this family risk factor depends on something that happened years before the disease made its appearance. They still don't know whether some form of shared susceptibility, some defective gene, or something in the environment is to blame for multiple sclerosis striking more than one member of a family, but they're sure the disease was not "caught" from a family member.

Aside from fearing contagion, some friends are simply uncomfortable. Some overexpress sympathy. Other people "tune out," one girl commented. "They say they don't want to bother me." As a patient as well as a psychologist, Dr. Uhlmann summed up the way many people with the disease feel about former friends:

"I felt uncomfortable about their being uncomfortable with me. It was almost as if I had leprosy. If I'd had a stroke or heart attack or cancer they could understand, but this was a fear of the unknown."

The decision to tell people you have the illness comes hard when you have no idea how friends will react. "Who's going to write on a Christmas card, 'I'm getting a wheelchair'?" Barbara McGrath asked. But when the wire services took her picture at the White House in her wheelchair as MS Mother of the Year, her friends sent the picture from one to another and now she is less reluctant to talk.

Ann Krasnicki says her boss at the CIA told her that "you've accepted the fact you have it when you can talk about it." She may not mention it on a first date, but she vows that if she ever gets married her husband-to-be will know as much about the disease as she does before they exchange vows. "I may not have another attack for twenty years," she said, "but I don't think it would be fair not to tell."

A woman who has had the disease for years said she always tells her friends because if she has a dinner party and tires, they understand she may have to go to bed early but she expects them to stay the evening and enjoy themselves. Another woman was having a dinner party for her son's fiancée. She had worked hard all day to make things right. Halfway through the meal, she had to excuse herself and go to bed. The startled girl, knowing nothing of her prospective mother-in-law's malady, thought she had done something very wrong. The girl was distressed, the family embarrassed, but they had asked for it. They had kept the illness secret and their little plot backfired.

One man I know says if somebody comes up to ask him why he uses two canes, he tells them he had a back injury. "I've shied away from admitting it because people get scared if you have a disease as opposed to an injury. No matter what you say, they think it might be contagious. Besides, I don't want to be treated any special way." Finally, surrounded by understanding friends, he is beginning to emerge from his cocoon of withdrawal. Another man said he regularly told anyone who asked about his cane that he had "this old football injury." When he tried that on his daughter, though, she said her mother—his estranged wife—had already told her he had multiple sclerosis.

Gerry Shur, my Justice Department friend, lifted a great weight from the shoulders of his son's band leader when he convinced him there was no stigma attached to the disease and he should tell people about it. Gerry said it was bad enough to carry the burden of the disease without the extra burden of concealment. The tremendous relief the band leader feels now is not only because the faculty and staff no longer suspects drinking is what makes him stagger. The attitude of the students has changed, too. Now, because he has told them the truth, they feel closer to him and grateful for the effort he exerts on their behalf.

One girl complained that when she told her friends they gradually abandoned her. She carefully explained all the things that might go wrong with the body; she made it sound so awful that her friends were frightened. After that, she advised fellow victims not to tell their friends or they would lose them, but she admitted that she had only told the negative things.

A group of people with multiple sclerosis who compared notes concluded they were the ones at fault. *They* were deserting their *friends*. When one woman felt bad, she would call her friends on the telephone and tell them so. She never called them when she felt good. And they drifted out of her life.

Dr. Jocelyn Gill developed a faithful following during her years with the space agency and used these friends to celebrate the good times of her life. A friend of hers told me that when Dr. Gill came out of an exacerbation, she had a "coming-out party" for her friends.

People with multiple sclerosis do have remarkably true friends. If it weren't for them, some people I know would be in nursing homes or housebound or forgotten by all but paid attendants. Friends have often pushed people with multiple sclerosis further on the road to hope than their own families have.

Norma Grimes had come home to die. She freely admits it. All she had strived for, the success she had achieved as a dental hygienist, her ambition to study dentistry—all of it was lost to multiple sclerosis. Her eyesight was failing and she could not use braille even if she wanted to because of the tremor in her hands. Her legs no longer held her up. In fact, she could not even sit up without bracing herself. She became totally dependent on her mother and young daughter for everything, even to cut a banana for her.

She had remained in bed a year and still she did not die. Every day she had to wake up to another day. She had become silent, noncommunicative, difficult to live with, hard to befriend. Two friends, though, refused to be rebuffed. They tried to get her interested in teaching good dental habits to schoolchildren. When she shook them off, they read up on her disease and became convinced she could be rehabilitated. They called the city's vocational rehabilitation office and the Multiple Sclerosis Society. Both sent representatives. With the help of her friends, they persuaded her to go to the Pittsburgh Guild for the Blind to learn to live with blindness and her disease.

Today Norma Grimes has her own apartment. She is doing everything for herself—from cooking to writing checks. It was her friends who got her out of bed. She said she had been "bringing them down with me. I said to myself, These people are interested in me and I'm not interested in myself. I've got to do something."

Bob Clark, the man of many trades, also is a man of many

friends. He had bought a chair glide to go upstairs when he could no longer walk, but had no way to get down the long flight of outside stairs. Either friends had to carry him or he would be doomed to being a prisoner in his own home. He designed what he needed, but the job would cost $1,900 and he had already spent his savings on the inside lift. He was trying to figure out how he could get a loan when friends stepped in. He is a Mason like his father before him, and around his lodge they say, "He's very close to us." He was close enough for them to put $500 toward the porch lift. The D.C. chapter of the Multiple Sclerosis Society matched it with $500; the chapter's patient services director, Diane Afes, put in her own $50 and got her friends to put in more. Clark's relatives and neighbors did the rest. When he tried to thank them, a neighbor reminded him, "Don't you remember a hot Saturday when you came home from work and found me with a truckload of soil dumped in my front yard? You pitched in and helped me haul it around to the back." Another neighbor recalled how Clark would prune their hedges.

All of them were there for the unveiling. They watched him ride the elevator to the ground. There were tears in his eyes as he thanked them. He can go to physiotherapy now, to the doctor, to the swim program, to lodge meetings without asking for help. His friends have given him the gift he prizes most—his independence.

A friend may have saved the life of a brilliant but almost wholly disabled man. He called the girl one day to tell her point-blank that he was going to end it all. "Oh, you can't now," she told him. "I just washed my hair. I don't have my face on. I can't come out like this, so you can't kill yourself yet." She promised to come over after a while, but as he waited for her, he realized how stupid he had been. "If she had not made light of it," he told me, "if she had gotten serious and acted like she thought I would do it, I might have done it." He has never again contemplated suicide.

Even less than intimates will rally around if they think they can be helpful. Gerry Shur discovered that while he was in the hospital a neighborhood friend called the Justice Department to find out what health benefits Shur had, and when they wouldn't tell him, he concluded Shur had none. He went to others in the neighborhood and asked if they would chip in $10 or $20 a month to keep the family going. The friends agreed to support him for an indefinite period. Shur learned about the offered help only by chance after he returned to work. If he had not been able to work, he would have been well covered by pension and insurance. The man's gesture, however, gave friendship another dimension.

Dorothy Jenkins, who had had the disease half a dozen years, was trying out a new van with her husband when he dropped dead of a heart attack. She had never been close to his family, her parents were dead, and she had no children. The shock of her husband's death put her in the hospital with a major attack. While she was recuperating her doctor suggested that she go into a nursing home. Instead, she returned alone to the big old house where she and her husband had lived. She knew she had to move, but where and how? Her friends took it from there. A friend in the real estate business found her a small one-story house. Other friends got her moved, put two months' worth of groceries in her freezer, and found her a van with a lift so she can get into it herself and take off. Without her friends, her future was in a nursing home.

Dr. Kathleen Shanahan Cohen remembers an incident— many years after her first bout with the disease—when she was determined to get to the Acropolis, despite brace and cane, up the long smooth slippery stones. She would not have made it if a Swedish engineer had not come along and said, "Seems to me you need some help." With that, he took her arm and hauled her to the top.

Michael Rubin, Department of Justice attorney, encountered another friendly stranger at a theater. The theater was not equipped especially for wheelchairs, so the chief usher escorted Michael and his wife to seats on the aisle and directed the ushers to seat everyone else in that row from the other side. One man came in late, and when he saw Michael in a wheelchair on the aisle, he coped without fuss. He asked people in the row behind his seat to get up so he could climb over. He made the over-the-seat trip during intermission, too. When Elaine Rubin thanked him, he told her, "My pleasure, I'm glad your husband could come to the theater."

Almost everyone I talked with wanted to tell me about a kind gesture, from the time a passing stranger picked a man up when he lay helpless on the ground to all the neighbors who regularly do the grocery shopping. Marilyn Pollin, marital and family therapist, calls friends "my support network," and Dr. Uhlmann says, "I find people are very helpful when you need them." Once when he fell in a government building and banged himself up a bit, he called a girl he knew on the next floor. "I fell. Do you have any Band-Aids in your desk?" Within two minutes, three women and two men were crowded around him. He looked at them and asked, "Does it take five people to bring one lousy Band-Aid?" One of them replied, "We heard you fell and we were concerned."

People with multiple sclerosis can use all the friends they can find because they have enough of what I call enemies. Certainly those who carelessly or callously pull them down or try to put stumbling blocks in their path can be thought of in no other way. Here are some on my enemy list:

A family was dining out and the mother with multiple sclerosis got up to go to the ladies' room. As she staggered, a man at a nearby table commented, "Look how stoned she is." The woman's husband got to his feet and tried to restrain his anger as he said, "That lady had only one drink. She has multiple sclerosis. I think you owe my wife and daughters an apology." The man muttered an apology to the young girls but the evening was ruined.

Lori Sanjiau's fingers mean everything to her as a musician; nevertheless one girl told her about an organist with multiple sclerosis who couldn't play any more because her hands trembled so. Another mentioned a pianist who had to stop playing because her fingers were numb.

Penny Renzi described an incident she cannot forget. A woman ran across a room and grabbed her and asked, "Are you all right?" When Penny said yes, the woman told her, "We were afraid you'd faint or something because of the way you walk."

"My first impulse was to sock her. Do you think that was a strange thing to do or am I strange to question it?" Penny asked me. I told her no she was not, but that she should understand that some people batten on the misfortunes of others. Those who ascribe noble motives to everyone contend that when people ask me why I limp, they are motivated only by genuine concern. The skepticism born of years of investigating makes me doubt that. I think they are just as often prying busybodies. Every person with multiple sclerosis who limps or uses a crutch or a cane or a wheelchair is constantly being asked why. Usually they are too polite or it would be too impolitic to say, "None of your business." They patiently answer the question over and over or make up reasons as my friends did—football injury, slipped disc, anything to get them off their back. I am playing with an answer which I offer free to others in need of one: "I hate to be immodest but I happen to have the disease of the brilliant, rich, and famous— multiple sclerosis!"

Eileen Quick, wife and mother, added another enemy. A new shopping center had made parking space available for the handicapped. One day when she parked there to pick up a cake, she heard the proprietor of the ice cream store telling a friend, "If I had a screwdriver and a pair of pliers, I'd take the handicapped parking sign down because it keeps business away from my store." Dr. Panzarella, Handicapped American of the Year in 1977, had a variation on the same theme. "All the disabled one wants is an opportunity to compete without added handicaps—like being ticketed after getting parking privileges."

Also in the enemy camp are people who use words like "crippled," "disabled," or "handicapped" to describe persons who still think of themselves as whole. A girl told of trying to take a midterm exam when her arm was shaking so badly that she could not even write her name. "I went up to the teacher," she said, "and asked if I could please have somebody write for me because I couldn't write. He called across the room, 'Ann, would you help this crippled girl, please?'" Until that moment, she had never thought of herself as crippled.

There are other enemies—employers who until recently, and even today if they can get away with it, fire or demote or fail to promote people with multiple sclerosis. One experienced worker told me that his employer continually reminded him how grateful he should be for his job and promoted a less experienced man over his head. My friend, at least, has the satisfaction of knowing that the man now theoretically his superior regularly comes to him for advice and assistance. A woman who had worked for an insurance company more than six years and had never taken a day's sick leave was fired as unsatisfactory after telling her supervisor about her multiple sclerosis. A woman manager of a fast-food store returned after an attack to be put on half pay, although she continued to work full time.

Police are supposed to befriend the helpless, but even they can become enemies. One of my friends was telling me that she had walked too far on her lunch hour without a cane. Noticing a patrol car passing, she hailed the policeman. Could he run her down to the next block because she had multiple sclerosis and she didn't think she could make it on her own? "Take a cab," the policeman replied brusquely and drove off. She had no money for a cab, so all she could do was cling to one parked car after another until she reached her office door. If she had noticed the policeman's number, she could have made trouble for him because his chief's sister has multiple sclerosis.

More than one insurance company has gone on my enemy list. There was the insurance company that refused to pay for a practical nurse's services, although the family's insurance seemed to cover them and the doctor had so prescribed. There was the insurance company that fired the girl with multiple sclerosis after six years of absence-free employment. And the big auto insurer that tried to cancel the policy of a man simply because he acknowledged that he had multiple sclerosis. The girl who lost her job had been fired too long ago for me to help, and I could not help the husband get a practical nurse for his wife either. But I *had* investigated auto insurance as a reporter and still had my contacts. When I told the insurance commissioner that the man's insurance had been canceled apparently because he put on his license renewal application that he had the disease and not because of any accident, the commissioner ordered a hearing and my friend won hands down.

Among other enemies are the charlatans who promise miracle cures and the so-called friends who make people with multiple sclerosis feel guilty for not trying cures that are always hundreds of dollars and miles away.

With so many enemies—and every person with the disease has met most of them at one time or another—they need all the friends they can muster.

Chapter 4

Love, Sex, Marriage, and Children

The marriage ceremony of one couple was rewritten at their request to say not "for better or for worse" but "I take you as you are." The bride had multiple sclerosis. As those who live with it know, multiple sclerosis takes the measure of love. If a marriage can survive our disease, it demonstrates enough strength to withstand any threat. Some loves wither at the first test while others seem to grow more vital, nourished by adversity. Whatever was true before becomes accentuated by a partner's illness.

In the marriage sweepstakes, however, I would predict the odds favor two groups. There are the long-married couples whose companionship tested over years of adjustment can take on more stress without faltering, and the newly married couples who faced the disease honestly and openly before they wed.

The motivations of the men who marry women with multiple sclerosis are many and mixed. Sometimes, the two have been longtime sweethearts and nothing is too big for them to face. Sometimes, a couple has already set the wedding date when the prenuptial excitement prompts the first symptoms to surface. This is a test some men fail. One mother had already sent out the invitations to the wedding when the man reneged.

When her daughter was wooed and won by another man several years later, the mother hesitated so long in sending out wedding invitations, not believing her daughter's good fortune, that some guests missed the wedding.

Sometimes a man marries a young woman in a wheelchair out of a mix of emotions, and none of them is pity. He can admire her spirit, her refusal to let the disease best her, her outgoing interest in helping others to live with similar problems. That was partially the motivation of a man I know who truly admired his lively fiancée. He also was impelled to take on this sizable added responsibility by the challenge of making a life for the two of them to share. And finally, he confided to a friend, "I need to be needed."

The girl who needed him had a gentleness about her that demanded nothing for herself. Her voice was soft as she spent her time making calls of reassurance to newly diagnosed patients. If she was worried about reaching her mid twenties without a true love, she never mentioned it, but her friends were concerned and one of them acted. She had her boyfriend arrange a double date, wheelchair and all. The blind date led to marriage, but not until she had proved herself. He had told her that he would do anything for her, but first she must try to manage for herself. Determined to show him he had not misplaced his faith, she refused to be pushed down the aisle to the altar. Instead, she climbed out of her wheelchair and walked down the aisle. "A miracle," her friends murmured. But it was not the only miracle that wedding day. At the reception, the groom asked the orchestra to play a slow waltz, then plucked his bride out of her wheelchair, placed her arms around his neck and, as she leaned against his chest, they slowly circled the dance floor together. The small town where all this happened will never get over that day.

Jewell Phillips, one of the young women I met at a multiple sclerosis "rap session," later told me she thought no one would be interested in her anymore when she started using a cane, but one man at her work was. Just before Christmas of 1976, he strolled over to her desk, stole a kiss, and invited her out to lunch. On their first date, he asked her to marry him. He confided that he had admired her for years. She responded by telling him about the disease. Undeterred, he continued to court her. When they went for blood tests, he asked to talk further with the doctor to learn how he could help her. "I love my marriage," Jewell says. "I didn't think it could happen but it did!"

Just as women with multiple sclerosis wonder if anyone will ever ask to marry them, men with the disease wonder if they should ask a woman to share their life and if they will be accepted if they do ask. Michael Rubin, the attorney at Justice, had a wife and child when the disease struck. Thereafter, he had neither. He took the divorce philosophically and buried himself in his legal work. When the doctor told him that a wheelchair might be better for him than stumbling around with a cane, he took that philosophically, too. "If I couldn't walk, I couldn't walk." The wheelchair led to Elaine.

She worked for a firm selling orthopedic appliances—a pert, pretty girl who could share Michael's easy laughter.

Michael reflected on what Elaine meant to him. "This illness makes you wonder whether you're still attractive to the opposite sex—was I a disability or was I still me." He was dating another girl at the time when he asked. She very honestly said yes, a wheelchair would bother her. Elaine simply answered, "Your wheelchair doesn't matter to me at all."

Elaine told me, "He's got his sickness on the outside where you can see it, but some men have it on the inside where you can't see it—and that's worse."

The wedding required considerable logistics. The rabbi, who had never performed a wheelchair wedding, was so flustered that he tripped over the wire for the tape recorder that Michael and Elaine used to record their wedding. Michael had to forgo the traditional *huppah*, or wedding canopy, symbol of home or bridal chamber in the Jewish faith, because the wheelchair took up so much space. The equally traditional breaking of the glass by the groom had to be done by the best man in a smashing finale. Only the rabbi had stood. The bride and groom sat, one in a chair decorated with white ribbons, the other in a wheelchair.

Just as architectural barriers that impeded the handicapped are slowly coming down, so are sociological and sexual barriers. Unconventional living arrangements are being accepted, and so is sexual experimentation. That may be a blow to Victorian views of sex, but it can be salvation to the handicapped, particularly the men who feel uncertain about their ability to perform and to satisfy. Most of the men either live with a girl or see several regularly. Some are divorced; others have never been married. But before they propose they want to be sure they can satisfy their partners' needs and their own. One young man told me his greatest satisfaction was in meeting and now living with a smart and perceptive girl who sees beneath his apparent well-balanced air of tranquility to an underlying bitterness, depression, and self-pity he succeeds in hiding even from himself. He wants to marry her, wants to have children with her, but he also wants to be sure he can make her happy. So he lives with her while he thrashes out his problems with a neurologist. A psychologist commented to me that he should be talking instead with a psychologist or marriage counselor because the problem that obviously worries him most is impotence and that, he says, is 90 percent psychological.

Even among the experts, opinion differs widely on how much of impotence is actually physical and how much is induced by a reluctance to experiment with sexual techniques or by an assumption that multiple sclerosis and impotence go together. I asked Dr. Kurtzke how much impotence was psychological. "For a given patient," he replied, "it's often difficult to tell, but ordinarily if one has no major bowel or bladder dysfunction, then the chances are great that he should not be impotent on a neurogenic basis in MS."

Dr. Simon Horenstein, chairman of the department of neurology in the St. Louis University School of Medicine, explained that multiple sclerosis does most of its spinal cord damage to the back of the cord; since the nerve mechanism affecting sexual function lies at the front of the spinal cord, it's likely to be spared. This, he said, applies particularly to the ability of men to attain an erection and perform sexually. The erections may be more fleeting, but the majority, he said, are capable of sexual intercourse. I personally know of two men with multiple sclerosis who each have had ten children.

A fellow professor at St. Louis University's School of Medicine, Dr. Harry Schoenberg, director of the division of urology, agreed that impotence is not a common problem in multiple sclerosis.

Most of the young men I talked with, from the newly married to the never married, emphasized that a woman means more to them now than simply sexual gratification. These men want rapport, understanding, companionship, as they never did before—not as a substitute for sex but as a recognition of the need to share a terrifying, sometimes overwhelming, problem.

Psychologists and marriage counselors also emphasize "pleasuring" a woman, but they refuse to concede that the man with multiple sclerosis cannot be pleasured, too. To make that possible, they often have to work their way through what psychologists consider an incredible amount of misinformation, frustration, and inhibitions. At a marriage session for people with multiple sclerosis and their mates, when one man suggested to another that he try masturbation, he replied that would be disloyal to his wife. Some couples had simply blanked sex from their minds until the marriage counselor warned them, "Sex is like annual leave. You either use it or lose it."

Dr. Dorothy Adler, a clinical psychologist, head of the pain clinic at the VA hospital in Washington, a VA consultant, and frequent speaker to multiple sclerosis groups, said she deals with the problem of impotence in men with the disease by taking the focus off intercourse as an exclusive goal, off performance alone. She tries to make them recognize that making love does not necessarily have to culminate in intercourse to be both satisfying and gratifying. It "takes the heat off" men to learn they can pleasure their spouses in other ways, through experimentation, trying to discover what pleases their mates, what is arousing to them.

Sigmund Freud, Dr. Adler said, did a great disservice in identifying only a few erogenous zones when there are actually many erogenous zones and they are unique from individual to individual. "Pressure points on the body are extremely sensitive—the inside of the wrist and the inside of the elbow. Many other points are also sensitive—the insides of the thighs, the temples. They may vary from person to person. The discovery of where your own are is part of the adventure.

"Even men who are totally impotent can derive a great deal of satisfaction from fondling, from handling, from massage, and they can certainly bring their partners to climax. They can really very much satisfy each other short of intercourse by pleasing their mates and by being pleased."

Dr. Adler teaches them to fantasize actively. "If they're good students, they actually experience orgasm in their minds." She suggests they imagine the sensations in their penis, how to simulate feelings of arousal. "Their spouse may be rubbing their stomachs or fondling their scrotum. In their mind, they can amplify the sensation, the fact they are lying together, their nakedness, their closeness, anything that serves to arouse them, whatever erotic imagery they are able to conjure up."

A kind of intimacy may be created that did not occur even with intercourse itself. "It's the essence of intimacy, the essence of sharing. Patients tell me physical intimacy was never the problem for them emotional intimacy was, that physical nakedness is easier to achieve than emotional nakedness."

The trouble with sex books, she complained, is that ultimately everything they teach has intercourse as its goal.

Impotence need not affect all men and it need not be permanent. If a man who is troubled by impotence relaxes thoroughly, knowing he is not expected to perform, he sometimes will be able to achieve erection and orgasm. "Once the demand requirement is removed and they don't have to worry about disappointing their partners, they are frequently able to achieve erection. There are times when such impotence is purely physiological, but sometimes there's a big psychological overlay. When all a man's energies are directed toward worrying about himself, being scared about himself, he has precious little energy left to devote to lovemaking. Maintaining depression takes a lot of psychic energy. Any emotional state—depression, anxiety—requires a lot of energy, so much energy that none is left for anything else."

Dr. Adler said she suggests ways a man with multiple sclerosis can escape the negative thoughts that rob him of his manhood. "If you teach them to have pleasurable thoughts and fantasies, what you're doing is extinguishing the feeling of failure and the concern of not performing. Just as feeling relaxed and feeling anxious are mutually exclusive competing responses, if they are anxious, there's no way they can be relaxed; if they are relaxed, there's no way they can be anxious."

Both Dr. Adler and Dr. Uhlmann, the psychologist-patient who spends much time advising fellow members of the multiple sclerosis community, endorse the reversal of the conventional sex positions. A man who spends most of his time in a wheelchair agreed: "When your stomach muscles and your leg muscles go, your wife can get on top."

Dr. Panzarella, a leading expert on the needs of the handicapped and himself a patient, stresses that the wife has to be willing to assume a more active role—"but this is part of a happy marriage. If a wife psychologically castrates a man, he's through and so is their marriage." He noted, though, that wives are more likely to remain with victims of multiple sclerosis than husbands to stay with wives with the disease.

The national divorce rate for all couples is now close to one out of two marriages. Divorces among couples where one is stricken with multiple sclerosis are said to be even more frequent. I doubt it myself. There are no statistics and the estimate is sheer guesswork. Among people I know with multiple sclerosis, many have stayed together. Among several who have been divorced or separated, a question arises each time: Would this marriage have become a divorce statistic even without multiple sclerosis? Did she marry him because he was obviously on his way to the top and would she have divorced him in any case if he failed to give her all she desired? Did he marry her because she roused sexual envy in his friends and would he have divorced her in any case when her looks faded with maturity and her middle thickened?

These are some of the contrasts I encountered among married couples:

One husband told me, "Changing catheters goes beyond what a husband is supposed to know or do, and I draw the line at the douches she has to have twice a week."

But Bill Dalton said that when his wife's catheter clogged up he would take her to the hospital. Until she was treated she would wait in great pain. Now, he prefers to care for her himself when a nurse is not available. A doctor explained to him how to change catheters, how to give enemas. "If the nurse isn't there, I do it and with far less trauma for her than a nurse." Rita relaxes with her husband, though she can communicate with him only with her eyelids.

This is a marriage of mutual strength. "She's given me the same support as if she hadn't had MS. The fact she's physically handicapped isn't important in our relationship. There's a lot of normal living if you don't let it get you down."

One husband took early retirement so he could be with his wife in case she needed him. He takes her to yoga classes and stays to learn the exercises so he can help her do them at home.

Yet another husband beats his wife. She is too helpless to escape him. Still another tells his wife he will take her to no more doctors because "the illness is all in her head." A group of patients hears a husband say, "If I want a dry bed tonight I've got to get home and take her to the bathroom." His wife was not there to hear that. Such husbands seem, fortunately, to be rare.

More are like this one: When a girl offered her husband a way out—a divorce—knowing how much he expected of a wife, he refused. She was more important to him than anything else. "I feel God was good to me in choosing my husband," she said.

Lucy Handler, wife of the president of the National Academy of Sciences, says her husband pushes her to do everything "we can squeeze out of the world for me to do. I react as well as I can."

Her husband put it more forcefully. "My role is never to let her quit, to be hard and cruel but never to let her quit." This "hard and cruel" man kept the truth of her disease from her for seven years because he felt if she really wanted to know what was wrong with her, she had all the knowledge she needed. Meanwhile, she lived a full and busy life, as she put it, "mother of a young and growing family, wife of a young and growing scientist."

She has repaid his years of coping alone with her illness in the best way she knew how. "The couple days in the hospital when I was paralyzed, I determined that only one of us was going to be paralyzed. I made my husband go to Russia that time without me and I lay there and read four volumes of the *Alexandria Quartet*. I made up my mind that he would go and do and be and if he let me come along for the ride, I would go, too, and that's what I have done. That wasn't nobility, just practicality."

Often the husband's attitude toward the disease is all the victim needs to live the full life. Without that, many women would fold, become uncared for and uncaring. My friend Lois Ryan said when she told her husband the diagnosis, he took it in a matter-of-fact way, as unexcited as if she were saying she had to have her appendix removed. His attitude— to face whatever has to be faced, "but let's not face it ahead of time." So they bicycled together as long as she could, switched to a tandem bicycle when solo riding became too much for her, and now exercise at the same health club. They are not looking ahead to borrow trouble.

Marilyn Pollin says she owes a great part of her psychological and physical well-being to her husband. "He refused to give up on me." Despite two canes and sometimes a walker, she not only works as a marital and family therapist but serves as senior staff supervisor at a mental hygiene clinic she helped found years ago and heads the Otto Rank Center, a new psychological organization.

The healthy husband can bolster a wife's shaken ego by offering convincing reassurance; he can cope with rambunctious youngsters; or keep his wife from doing too little or too much. He can also step into the part of substitute homemaker. When Elaine Dewar had an attack, her husband worked at home in the mornings to fix breakfast and prepare lunch. While she was sleeping, he would put the children in the playpen beside her bed and give the baby her bottle. Debbie, the two-and-a-half-year older sister, would take the bottle away when it was empty.

When Elaine seemed tired he would suggest that she take a nap and he would start dinner. "When we first got married, it was clear that he was brought up to think the wife did wifely things. Now he's a better cook than me."

Eileen Quick, a lively blond, said she tends "to shy away from people because I don't want to be a 'burden.'" When she retreats, her husband buoys her. "People like you for what you are, not because you have MS or are a little disabled." When she confronts him with "I don't want you to feel sorry for me; I want you to be here because you want to be here and because you love me," he simply replies, "I wouldn't be here if I didn't want to be. If the roles were reversed and I was the one who had health problems, where would you be?" Because Jack Quick, who raised a family before he lost his first wife to cancer, empathizes with Eileen's problems, her own two daughters are learning to understand her better (her first marriage had ended in divorce). "He can talk to the children better than I can, because he's once removed. He's sort of a buffer and can make the children realize they have to push a little more, do a little more than their friends."

Like other thoughtful wives I encountered, Eileen refuses to take love for granted. She works at it by establishing "quality time." She and her husband picked up the phrase from a sermon on the quality of life. Quality time is time together, away from the children, from friends, from domestic arguments, a regular time noted on the calendar. If anybody calls, they are busy. She plans the day, sets the stage with candlelight, the best silver and china, flowers, music on the stereo, and dresses for dinner.

The children share the fun of planning and then leave them alone together after an early dinner of their own, going to their own rooms for the evening. "We don't talk politics or bring up any controversial topics, no family financial discussions, no heavy decisions," Eileen said. "Our quality time is too precious."

Jack had refused to believe she had multiple sclerosis before they were married because she showed no outward sign of it. He assumed that everyone with the disease was like his mother, wheelchair-bound. He found it hard to believe that Eileen had pain because his mother had no pain, and he thought victims were spared pain. He knows now that cramped muscles sometimes do breed pain and that the disease never affects two people in exactly the same way.

Penny Renzi and her husband, Colonel Eugene Renzi, learned together to keep down stress in their household. Sometimes that is easier said than done with a household of teen-agers. "He's terrific, really my rock. He helps by minimizing the things that should be minimized, any problems with the children or school. His attitude is that it will be all right, that there's always an answer. I tend to get uptight. He's always the calm one, so then I am, too."

The closeness of twenty years of marriage helps her now. It hit her hard when a member of her wedding party—one of the three who later came down with multiple sclerosis—was divorced. "How horrible to go through multiple sclerosis and then face getting divorced." Her husband left her with the two children they had adopted.

When Pauline Schultz knew this was the man she wanted to marry, she told him she had multiple sclerosis and, like the good nurse she was, she gave him all the information she thought he would need to make a decision—despite the doctor she had dated earlier who told her he would have married her if it had not been for the disease. (At the time she had retorted that she would never marry a doctor.) Now they discussed her illness together in scientific terms, the statistical probability of her winding up in a wheelchair. At her suggestion, he visited her physician to discuss her problems, and he still wanted to marry her. "I wasn't keeping anything from him. It would be the basis for a good solid marriage."

And it has been. "I don't have to go to a psychiatrist. I can cry on my husband's shoulder because we share. The MS is not just mine. It's the whole family's problem in many respects because we all have to live with it." As her two girls have gotten big enough to understand, she has taught them how to function without her. Her husband has no qualms about stepping into her role whenever needed—cooking dinner, vacuuming the house, marketing. "He's got the emotional security to do it."

Some marriages founder simply because a man lacks the self-confidence to play housekeeper and even nurse occasionally for his ailing wife, but as Pauline said, when a man has emotional security, he can do it all. Jean Urciolo used a similar description of her own husband. "He's extremely secure. He knows he's very good at what he does so he can give me the help I need. John is always there to help. When he saw me carrying a laundry basket down the steps, he said, 'Why should you do that? I can do it.' " She is grateful to him, too, for keeping her illness a secret from her long enough for her to finish school. "I know I'm extremely lucky."

Jacqueline du Pre, the great cellist stricken by multiple sclerosis, has used those same words repeatedly to interviewers in talking about her husband. The beautiful blond cellist and Daniel Barenboim, the noted pianist and conductor, were married in Jerusalem after touring there in concert during the

1967 Middle Eastern War. They had everything—youth, exciting talent, good looks, and their love. She had played across the world to wildly enthusiastic audiences. He was much in demand also. They often appeared together, as a duo or with him conducting and her soloing.

The future could not have been more golden when it started turning gray. She had brushed aside episodes of double vision and aches and pains but now her arms were getting heavy and her eyes were drooping with drowsiness. Then the strength and feeling in her fingers began to go. On January 15, 1973, she played the last concert with her husband in New York's Philharmonic Hall, and before the end of the next month, she had given her last performance.

When she went into a London hospital for tests and was told flatly that she had multiple sclerosis, he was giving a concert series in Israel. Deciding not to tell him the truth and make his concert tour more difficult, she called to report what the doctors had said, but kept the verdict from him. He called the hospital himself to get the truth (from her doctors), talked with doctors in Israel about what multiple sclerosis could mean to his wife, then he flew home without letting her know he was on the way.

"He just stood there at the door and said, 'Hello,' in a voice that had all the love in the world in it.

"It was such a wonderful gift for him to give me because Danny is completely dedicated to music. He never misses concerts. He'd canceled his remaining concerts to fly back to me."

That was no one-night stand. Dan Barenboim learned how and did cook until he found a housekeeper who adores music. He arranged to live in a house that had been built for a disabled person; she could be wheeled into an elevator from her upstairs bedroom and reemerge in the downstairs hall. His presents to her are thoughtful, like the bed tray, with side pockets for her mail, that can be propped up as a book rest because her hands—the hands that once had the power to exert twenty pounds of pressure for a single note—now lack the strength to hold a book for long. He is said to have turned down the directorship of the New York Philharmonic to be with her, and when he goes to Paris to conduct the Orchestre de Paris, he calls her each night. When she confesses to fears that he might weary of a no longer active partner, he reassures her with "I love you."

The wives of stricken husbands are not all perfect and neither are their husbands. One woman went back to work when her husband's tremors and semiblindness prompted him to stay home. She assured him in my presence that she would never leave him, and she did not. *He* left *her,* went home to his wealthy father and he then proceeded to sue her for alimony. An erstwhile friend said that young man gave multiple sclerosis a bad name. Another man left his wife of many years because her condescending attitude upset him so much that he was constantly falling, a reaction to stress. "She was as frightened about my illness in terms of *her* future, as I was about the unknowns of *my* future."

Some men, considering their disease an admission of weakness, want to keep it within the family circle. One, refusing to ask any form of help from neighbors or even from his brother-in-law, made his wife climb up on the roof to patch a leak rather than share his problems with the outside world. When the wife of another victim told her that she should set limits or she would be caught in a trap, the couple talked it over and decided to let the brother-in-law care for the roof.

Some men choose the path of nobility and offer their wives their freedom whether they want it or not. One wife told me that her husband sat her down and said if at any time she were to fall in love with somebody else, she should simply tell him and he would pack up and disappear forever. At first, she was devastated that he even had to think such thoughts, but then she accepted his response as a normal reaction to the illness. "I told him, 'I thank you very much for the gift of my freedom if I want it. I don't want it, but I will love you forever for it.' We said all these beautiful valiant things and got them out of the way. Now we're getting on with living our marriage."

John Kramer's wife told him during our conversation that multiple sclerosis has confirmed the fact that he is her best friend in addition to being her lover. Gerry Shur used almost the same words in describing his marriage. "My wife is not only my lover but my best friend," Shur said. "We had a step up when we had this crisis. A good marriage gets better because you can dismiss the unimportant things. We got over little garbage-type arguments. What was important was that we still loved each other; we still had our children; we could still communicate, could still give and feel love. Whether I was ten minutes late became less important, whether dinner wasn't done well had no importance. We weren't the least bit interested either in what a neighbor thought or did—just in what we did and could do together."

Because Miriam Shur is a clever wife, she will arrange for rest periods for her husband that he never suspects. If they are shopping and planning to go out in the evening she will decline to stroll around the shopping center because she has things she must do at home. Translated, that means he has a few hours to sit down and rest before they go out.

Shur believes firmly in the value of communications in cementing marriage, particularly an MS marriage. "If a patient doesn't say to his spouse, 'My legs are bothering me today,' he becomes irritable and the spouse doesn't understand why. It's much better to say, 'Something's bothering me. I think it's MS today and I'll have to take it easy.'" There are times, though, when even he thinks some thoughts should be kept to himself; he knows his wife is the same way. "As honest as a husband and wife are with each other, they can still fool one another into a little happiness."

The couple married the longest of any I interviewed also was the couple with the most disabled partner. Thirty-four years after their marriage, Mrs. Panzarella says, "I told him he was as normal as the next one."

He responds, "She didn't make me feel I was different. She always made me feel I was the father, the head of the family."

"The children always deferred to him," his wife says. "They knew he was the one they had to answer to."

She helps him in such a quiet, unassuming way that nobody notices it unless he calls attention to her himself. He was making a speech on breaking down barriers that face the handicapped one day when he suddenly paused, "I've got to stop a minute. My wife's arm is getting tired." Until he said it, probably few had noticed that she was holding a microphone to the mouth of her husband in his wheelchair.

When I asked Dr. James Q. Simmons of the National Multiple Sclerosis Society if he thought people with this disease should marry, he answered rhetorically. "Statistics reveal that a large proportion of MS patients never become seriously incapacitated, so why should they not marry?" Naturally, he said, a man or woman considering marriage should read the literature about the disease and ask a physician for up-to-date information about the course of remissions and exacerbations and what patient care might be needed if exacerbations become severe.

"Marriage to MS patients," said Dr. Simmons, "requires love, loyalty, understanding, patience, selflessness—the qualities needed but often lacking in all marriages."

Is multiple sclerosis hereditary? All the figures say no. Out of hundreds of thousands of people with multiple sclerosis, the disease is shared by parent and child less than 5 percent of the time. Genetic factors of some importance may be involved, but, current research reasons, they must be subjected to powerful environmental influences to develop into multiple sclerosis. What these influences are remains a mystery.

Some know-nothing relatives warn that pregnancy would surely precipitate an attack of multiple sclerosis. Others predict a dire fate for the babies. Dr. Horenstein says flatly: "Labor will not bring on an attack of multiple sclerosis. Labor will only bring on a baby." Authorities say a mother's multiple sclerosis poses no significant risk to the fetus.

The girls I talked to told me they never felt better than when they were pregnant. One girl said she wished she could be pregnant all the time because she felt so well then. She nearly made it. She had four children. Doctors are inclined to believe that body changes women usually experience during pregnancy are responsible for that feeling of well-being.

Researchers at NINCDS confirmed, however, what I had been told, that following delivery attacks may increase, "so effects tend to balance themselves out."

Advisors usually don't encourage women with multiple sclerosis to have children, but if they and their husbands want a family very much and can afford it financially and emotionally, they do not discourage them either. On the practical side, they're advised to use a formula service and disposable diapers and, if possible, to hire a housekeeper or at least a part-time helper around the house. An environment in which the new mother may be chronically exhausted, riddled with anxieties, and likely to lose her balance is hardly ideal for raising a child. Nevertheless, even a cautious advisor backed one such woman when she wanted to adopt a baby, arguing that the disabled would-be mother and the abandoned child would be good for each other as long as the couple could afford full-time help.

Some physicians tell their patients to go on the pill or get sterilized. Dr. Horenstein doesn't go nearly that far. "As a matter of good practice," he said, "it seems to me that a patient with multiple sclerosis who has been having a lot of recent difficulty should not take on an additional physical or emotional responsibility. I do not believe there is any reason for saying that a patient with multiple sclerosis who is otherwise well or has been stable for several months or years should not conceive and bear children if that is her choice."

None of the men and women I interviewed expressed any reservation about having children. As for the children, they may complain about doing more chores than other youngsters but they get to see their parents more often and seem to add stability to the marriage.

The marriages that work seem to follow a definite pattern, whether they are first marriages or second, whether the marriage occurred long before one was stricken or after learning about the illness. And in that pattern lies the hope for saving marriage despite the disease, for having children and enjoying as rewarding a relationship as any other married pair.

The pattern simply involves almost total honesty, sharing, and open lines of communication. If both parties to the marriage are fully aware they simply have one more load to carry, the shared load makes the good life possible. This is far from theory alone. I have drawn on my friends' experience for tips on how to make such a marriage work.

• An argument can bring a harmful physical reaction or, conversely, joyful occasions can pay off in greater strength, greater ability to perform.
• Try to avoid encumbrances to romance; if they must be there, make a playful joke of them. Keep your bedroom as nonclinical as possible.
• Initiate romantic occasions, such as candlelight and champagne in a bedroom. You are seeking to preserve the magic, mystery, and mystique of your love.

• If you are the healthy partner, avoid treating her or him always as handicapped, and never as more handicapped than she or he actually is.

• Whenever you call at work, never ask the person who answers how your husband or wife seems today. That simply reminds others of physical problems your spouse may want to downplay.

• Never argue in the bedroom or the car.

• You can help by teaching your partner when to say no to demands for his or her services.

• Never let the victim fear rejection if he or she should get angry or irritated. Anger and irritation are normal reactions, and your handicapped spouse should be urged to show feelings honestly so the other can be honest, too. Constantly strive for a normal life but recognize that at times the person with multiple sclerosis will be unable or unwilling to communicate. The door may be closed then, but only temporarily unless you press. Then you could have a full-fledged but unnecessary misunderstanding.

• Assure your spouse that he or she is no less a person when accepting help from others, including you.

• If you are the disabled one, do not expect your spouse always to be with you and you alone. You did not monopolize his or her attention before this happened, why do it now? Your mate needs time away from you to make the time with you more agreeable. Make your home a place of love, not a prison.

• Join other couples in a night on the town when you are well enough to enjoy it. Even sometimes when you feel less than tiptop, you should push yourself to a theater evening. You may be surprised to find how well you sleep after a change of scene.

• If your spouse is willing, the two of you might benefit from a Multiple Sclerosis Society meeting with couples like you—others who are trying to cope with the problems that sometimes get you down.

• You may not be able to play ball or tennis with your son or daughter but you can watch them play, cheer their progress, even correct their technique. You can take them to many sports events because sports arenas—like many theaters—now have special seating for the handicapped and sometimes half-price tickets. Particularly if you are a father, your disease is no excuse for shortchanging your children, but never say yes to something special unless you really plan to go.

• Keep the door to communications always open wide. When you cannot talk freely to each other, you are diminished and so is your love.

The suggestions that follow are aimed at wives of victims:

• Learn when and how to take the initiative without robbing him of his ego. You might even seduce him, not because you think he is afraid to test his abilities but as a way to demonstrate your love.

• If he finds it difficult to reach a dining area at work, fix lunch for him to take. Probably, he would rather "brown-bag" it than ask someone to fetch lunch for him.

Here are a few tips for husbands of victims:

• When your wife complains of being terribly tired, believe it. She may look fine but she has to stop whatever she may be doing and rest. This is no time to bring your boss home for dinner.

• If you cannot afford a cook, learn to cook yourself. Her friends will be glad to help out with their specialties until you get the hang of it. With frozen foods and other prepared meals, cooking is no big deal.

• If you have young children, convince your wife they will be better off in a day-care center where they can be looked after by professionals during the day so that when they come home she will be rested enough to play with them before bedtime.

I had planned to include tips on how to explain the disease to your children until I was told repeatedly that kids do not need a lot of explanation. I know that is true of kids I have encountered. Once, before I knew I needed a cane, I was stranded on a cobblestone street in a Mexican town and I knew I could never cross it without help. Since I had no Spanish, I made gestures to a small boy. He gave me a wide grin and his arm and we marched across the street together.

"Kids understand a lot more than adults," Dr. Uhlmann told me. "My youngsters have read and talked to me about MS. When my brother brought his two small girls here for a visit, we took them to the space museum and other points of interest, but when I asked them at the airport, as they were leaving, what was the best part of their visit, they both said, 'Wheeling you around in your wheelchair, Uncle Frank.'

"They are perceptive, too. When I told my kids I was sorry I couldn't teach them to ski, they said, 'Okay, you can't do that but you are always around to rap with.' They understand a heck of a lot more than we give them credit for, regardless of age."

When he had to go to the hospital but hesitated to go, his daughter said she would give up her planned trip to Denver unless he went to the hospital as he should. She packed his bag and tucked in a homemade valentine, now pasted on his window.

> While you are at the hospital, feeling kind of sick,
> Just remember to do one thing and that's to get well quick.
> Please try hard not to get depressed,
>   just remember to avoid all stress.
> The nurses will try to give you pills around the clock
> But just stick up for yourself, tell them you're the doc.
> I know that I will be going away, but my love for you is a feeling
>   that will stay.
> Just remember I'm your No. 1 fan
> Try not to forget you're my No. 1 man.
> Just remember I love you very much, too,
> And do me a favor and get well soon. Love, Wendy.

One day when Gerry Shur was sitting at home after his first attack, blinded, miserable, feeling sorry for himself, his teen-age daughter, Ilene, said, "Daddy, you have talked to us for so long about how we're supposed to act when we have a problem. You're not acting that way. Tomorrow when I come home from school, we're going for a walk."

The whole next day, Shur was terrified. He hoped she'd forget about the venture. But she didn't. Instead, she said, "Okay, daddy, it's time to go."

Shur remembered, "She put her arms out. I couldn't see. She touched me, I touched her. We locked arms and we started walking down the block. I'd hear kids saying, 'Hello, Mr.

Shur,' and I'd say hello back. I'm thinking there's a big world
out there where it's still Mr. Shur, still daddy. She described
what the day was like. It was bright. I could feel that it was.
Neighbors came over to say how nice it was to see me. That
walk with my daughter got me going again." He went back
to work a week later.

It was fortunate that Shur had sat his son and daughter
down and explained to them in terms they could understand
what the disease was all about, because one day in her health
class his daughter heard the teacher say of multiple sclerosis,
"That's the disease that turns people to stone." It could have
been terrifying for the child if her father had not briefed her
about the disease. As it was, she came home and told him the
teacher did not know what he was talking about.

Jeane Hofheimer said one of her sons told her as he lifted
her into the car: "Mother, you carried us for a long time. It
won't hurt us to carry you now." And Dr. Shanahan Cohen
could trace back the compassion that has prompted her son to
become a rabbi to the days when he would gulp back the embarrassment of carrying a woman's pocketbook because she
could not carry it herself.

Not that the children are angels of mercy all the time. The
youngsters of the handicapped usually have more chores to do
than other kids on the block and, naturally, they resent it at
times. Yet they do the chores without too much protest, often
with laughter and even with expressions of concern. I was still
new to the world of multiple sclerosis when a rap session was
held in my apartment. Brenetta Payne's young daughter,
Debbye, stayed inconspicuously in the background while the
talk swirled about her, but when I got up to bring in coffee
to the group, she was beside me instantly to help with the
cups and saucers, the cream and sugar. Nobody prompted
her. She was just there. Helping someone with a handicap was
as much a part of her life as studying for exams. I was not

surprised when Brenetta brought me her daughter's school essay headed, "My Mother Has MS."

Last summer, when my mother had her attack I told my friends that she "was sick" or "her leg hurts." I couldn't bring myself to tell them she had MS. This was largely because I myself didn't know what it was. I just knew that it turned my beautiful mother with a nice shape and plenty of boy friends into a 100-pound woman, who could no longer pass for 18.

I hated to see this change because I knew my mother remembered herself the way I did. During the month or two after her attack, I tried in every way to help her. I got angry when she would refuse my help and say, "I can do it." I wanted to walk for her. At times I didn't believe she couldn't walk; I just couldn't see how anyone could just NOT walk!

During this time, I brought her her food but I could see that she wished she could do it herself. My mother, the normally independent woman, relying on her 14-year-old daughter for everyday things.

My mother used to hide it from me, when her hand would shake, or when she suddenly stumbled in the street. I guess I was too young then.

I wish I could say that my mother got her strength and courage from me and my help but she didn't. She got it from her daily prayers to the Lord. And her walks with Him. She might not have been able to walk in our apartment, but she walked and still walks with Him in her mind and soul.

For people with multiple sclerosis, an understanding love makes the present more livable, but children are their hope for the future.

Chapter 5

The Blessed Therapy of Work

A research chemist in Akron, a construction engineer in Los Angeles, a jazz musician in Chicago, a private duty nurse in Woodbridge, Connecticut—multiple sclerosis has not stopped them. The chemist has had one patent published and four more applied for. The engineer specializes in space ventilation for the Los Angeles Department of Water and Power. The musician, a pianist with the Chicago Pops orchestra, has accompanied the top singing stars, although occasionally his hands and arms are cramped and his vision blurred. The nurse finds work the best medicine.

When multiple sclerosis strikes and maybe strikes again, when victims first get the verdict, they face the first and often most difficult decision: Should I go ahead and get my degree, should I finish my training, should I change jobs, change professions? While an employer, a professor, a wife, can be important in the decision, ultimately a person's own strength and own determination make the difference.

A man in his twenties was traveling in a wheelchair before he completed his Ph.D., but he reached it mainly because his advisors provided such strong backing and arranged for him to shine in public appearances. After one speech before a scientific group in Washington, he wound up with a good job

at the Environmental Protection Agency. In contrast, one
woman who had just completed her Ph.D. in physics was
advised by her mentor not to try for the job as a physicist for
which she had been training so long, because it might prove
too much for her. Friends at the Multiple Sclerosis Society
are now trying to repair the damage that man did.

In 1966, Gerry Shur was becoming involved in gathering
intelligence about organized crime. When multiple sclerosis
hit his eyes and his legs and pricked his body relentlessly with
pins and needles, he thought he was going to die but he never
thought he would not go back to work. At first when he
returned, his immediate superior, Jack Keeney, later number-
two man in the Justice Department's criminal division, would
"just happen" to be down at his end of the long corridor and
drop in to see if he would be interested in a certain criminal
investigation. Instead of summoning him as young attorneys
were always summoned, Henry Peterson, then chief of organized crime and racketeering, would find an excuse to stop
by Shur's office.

"They kept finding interesting things for me to do. They
would hang out a laundry line of work for me and let me pull
off anything I chose. Sometimes, my secretary had to read it
to me, because my quadruple vision had only gotten down to
double vision—but I was working. While they were making
excuses to come to my office, I started coming to them just
to let them know I could do a full day's work, that I was
the same guy I used to be."

They continued to be protective, however. When Shur accompanied his chief to testify before a congressional committee on organized crime, Peterson suggested that they take a
taxi back to the Justice Department, nearly a mile away. Shur,
knowing Peterson liked to walk, counter-suggested that they
walk since the day was so fine.

"When we got back to the department, Henry went to his

office and I went to mine and almost passed out, but I was absolutely delighted. I could do it!"

Within three years, Shur had regained enough strength to start arranging new lives and identities for those who risked death to testify against the Mafia.

Now, as attorney in charge of the Organized Crime Intelligence and Special Services Unit (the witness-relocation program), Shur works fourteen to sixteen hours a day, nights and weekends, because "my hobby and my occupation are the same," and in the last twelve years, he has not missed a day's work because of multiple sclerosis. He has to adjust to pins-and-needles assaults on his body, to blinking eyes, and sometimes overwhelming fatigue, but he has no intention of retiring. "Whatever your state," he said, "you will make it better if you say, 'I'll be damned if I'll surrender to this. To hell with it!' "

Although Gerry Shur believes in telling employers and associates quite frankly that he has multiple sclerosis, he does not make a practice of broadcasting it to strangers. One day a criminal seeking sanctuary was telling Shur his troubles. He said his wife had multiple sclerosis and went on to describe her problems. Obviously, he had no understanding of the disease or had not listened to the explanations offered by her doctor, so Shur explained the disease to him. An hour later, he called from the airport where he had gone to fly to his wife's side.

"How do you know so much about multiple sclerosis?" the fleeing criminal wanted to know.

"I have it," said Shur.

On another occasion, a witness who had been railing against the government began to complain about a chronic disease that bothered a relative. "But why tell you? You don't know what it's like." Shur just let him talk, but at that moment, he could not lift his left leg and his right hand felt as though somebody had been sitting on it for a month. Whenever things get bad, Shur picks up the miniature sole of a hiking boot he keeps on his desk or a toy replica of his trailer. They are symbols of what he can still do. He and his wife, Miriam, have bought a trailer for travel and taken up mountain climbing. There are handicaps. He gets tired, "but if I tire on a mountaintop, we pitch a tent and go to sleep." It was a greater achievement, he says, to overcome his fear of snakes than of multiple sclerosis.

The law can be a good profession for people with multiple sclerosis because cases can be tried sitting down. Several of my lawyer friends go to court in wheelchairs and even face the jury seated. Michael Rubin, one of three Justice Department attorneys I know of with multiple sclerosis, tries cases from his wheelchair and calls himself "the luckiest guy in the world" because he does the job he wants to do and feels successful doing. "The greatest thing in the world is to be looked up to by people who do the same thing you do. The lawyers I work with ask me questions. They are my so-called ego trip. They make me feel worthwhile."

People with multiple sclerosis are supposed to avoid stress, but one lawyer I know thrives on the stress of his working days. "As a computer analyst, I have to think fast on the job but I am very confident. I am in control." Stress on the job bothers him not at all, but when he is at home with the everyday problems of wife and family, his evening is ruined by double vision.

The jobs my friends are doing, the jobs they are determined to keep, may vary in prestige and power but they will fight to save them. They may deny, deny, deny that anything is wrong. They may give up a social life to stay strong enough for a working life. They may grab a nap instead of a lunch. And they may plow through snow when even a healthy person would hesitate to venture out, just to prove something to themselves, if not to anybody else.

Like Timothy Drury, the Buffalo prosecutor who battled drifts through Buffalo's worst snowstorm to reach court, Jean Ballard reported to her job at the Agriculture Department in Washington through a snow so deep I was amazed to reach her there—by telephone, of course. I would never go out in that kind of weather myself. How did she do it? She laughed and said her husband had told her repeatedly that it would not interfere with her goal of working every day if she stayed home this time, like all sensible people. "But I've got this thing about really trying to be here as much as possible. I think I have it within me." She wasn't doing the driving but she was so nervous during the two-hour drive through the snow and ice she could feel "numbness and tingling all over."

Jean Ballard had gone through everything—the dizziness, lack of coordination, blacking out; months in bed; three intervals in the hospital, being tested for a brain tumor that, of course, was not there; lying in the nurse's office crying because she had worked so hard and did not think she could make it.

Her new boss, the regional director of the Agriculture Department's audit division, had told her he would take a chance on her as his personal secretary because her work was so good. She was determined to prove him right. Her goal was to make it to work every day, and she kept it up for thirty-one weeks. "I used the work as therapy," she said. "I probably worked harder because I was so miserable. I had no time to think about myself. I had eighteen people working under me—four secretaries, the mail room, and the typing pool, all relying on me for information about their job."

A year from the December of her tears, her boss, in a formal evaluation, called her the best secretary he ever had. "I was beside myself with joy. It was like an extra reward. For a while there, when I couldn't get up and go to his office, he would come out here to my desk. I didn't know how long he would give me, but, as it worked out, I didn't let him down and I didn't let myself down. Today, he would have understood if I hadn't come to work through the snow but I couldn't let me down. I have these goals. . . ."

For Nancy Lewis, it was the combined demands of a job she loved, a home, a marriage, and three children that forced her to face the realities of her illness. She had climbed steadily on her job since she started in 1970 as a $6,500-a-year library technician in the Library of Congress. A few years ago, she noticed that her legs sometimes felt almost too heavy to lift; she had numbness and a prickling sensation, and she fell occasionally. But she pushed these things out of her mind. A doctor urged her to go into the hospital for tests, but she was pregnant and that was no time for tests. She worked up to two weeks before her son was born in January 1977, and three months later the doctor told her she had multiple sclerosis.

She accepted the verdict intellectually but emotionally continued to deny it, refusing to consider all the changes she would have to make in her life and probably should already have made. She continued to juggle a dozen chores, from cooking and caring for the baby when help was not available to driving her daughters to music classes where twelve-year-old Jenny played the violin in the county's prep orchestra and ten-year-old Leslie was starting on the flute. When she returned to work on a three-day-a-week schedule, she was exhausted before she ever reached her desk after the ride on the train from her suburban home and the long walk to the nearest taxi to take her to the library. Even with two Lofstrand crutches, she was dragging.

In January 1978, Nancy Lewis—by now promoted to assistant section head of the American-British exchange section, which collects all official documents of the British Commonwealth—had to go back to the hospital. For the first time, alone with an intravenous needle in her arm and the corticosteroid ACTH, used to combat acute attacks, working on her, Nancy squarely faced her disease. She talked it all over with her husband. He was reassuring. Yes, there had to be a real sharing of tasks. Yes, the baby would have to be placed with a baby-sitter every day whether she was home or not. Yes, she had to find some other way to get to work besides that tiring train ride.

When she came out of the hospital, she carried out the new life plan they had worked out together. The girls were given a deeper understanding of their mother's illness and the tasks assigned to them. It was hard to give up some of the time she had spent with the baby, but her son was getting to be too much for her to handle alone. Finally, a friend from the library offered to drive her to work, her husband's new job was nearby, and the rearrangement of her life was complete.

Joanne Bell and Jean McLean, the two young women with multiple sclerosis who work for the House Interstate and Foreign Commerce Committee, cope with the demands of rigorous jobs. Jean types the minutes of meetings of the full committee and five of its six subcommittees along with performing other committee chores, while Joanne's job is the committee calendar, keeping track of more than two thousand bills going through the committee each session of Congress. Although she was off the job for three weeks when the disease struck in 1977 with total fatigue and the full panoply of numb, tingling terror, it never occurred to her not to return. What did occur to her as her fingers refused to hit the right keys was that she would extend her duties into data management. She began to find out what programs were available from the House computer center, evaluating the work the committee needed, and putting the two together. She is planning now to take the training she needs. What she has going for her day to day are an understanding boss and fellow workers who know as much about multiple sclerosis as she does because she told them all. One girl in the office even thanked her for making it so easy for them to understand. "Because I feel comfortable with it," Joanne said, "I make my friends feel comfortable."

Joanne and Jean compare notes about how one or the other may be faring, but neither lets multiple sclerosis dominate her life. They have the second busiest committee on the House side of the Capitol so neither has time to rest the way she probably should. Joanne tries to get to the nurse's first-aid room once or twice a week to lie down during her lunch hour but rarely makes it. Jean escapes occasionally into the ladies' room when the noise becomes too much for her in the busy office and she can put her feet up to relax a few minutes during her eight-to-nine-hour day. She is grateful that 1976 is behind her. It was in 1976 that the disease returned after twenty-three years, then that she learned for the first time she had had it all along. Her arms and her legs were so weak and heavy she had trouble driving home. Now she tells herself her tiredness is no more than anyone else gets after a long day. Like Joanne, she forgoes weekend dates to recharge herself.

The majority of victims are still getting around, many years after being stricken, but for some the disease progresses to wheelchairs and ultimately to retirement. A determined person can postpone that day for years and Dr. Jocelyn Gill was more determined than most. Internationally and lovingly known as "the den mother of the astronauts" for her work in briefing the space men, she had lived with multiple sclerosis most of her life because her mother had it before her and she considered herself lucky, in a way, because she was spared the usual agonizing self-diagnosis of so many others with the disease. It hit her in 1945 when, armed with a master's degree in astronomy and astrophysics, she had begun teaching at Smith College. Mt. Holyoke College and Yale University fol-

lowed and, with her new Ph.D., she went to Arizona State
College to teach in Flagstaff's high, dry, and temperate climate. Regular swimming in the college pool kept the disease
at bay. In 1960 she could still drive across the country and
even shovel snow. Joining the National Aeronautics and Space
Administration, she began a new career of promoting scientific
exploration of outer space.

Until 1966 she was driving to work and managing without
help, a cheerful woman with prematurely white hair, but that
year, although her eyes were fixed on the stars, she had to face
a reality of the earthbound—crutches and braces. That was,
nevertheless, an up year for her. She was one of six women out
of the many thousands in the career government service to win
the Federal Woman's Award. And the recognition had nothing to do with her by now longtime multiple sclerosis. I
know, because I was on the board of trustees for the Federal
Woman's Award. When she was nominated by NASA for the
award, no mention was made of the disease. I was sure I
would have noticed it because that was the year I was finally
told that I had it, too; but to be certain now that hers was not
a pity award, I checked with the Civil Service Commission.
No, she was nominated for the award because she was great.
Another award the same year, however, *was* directly due to
the disease. Vice-President Hubert Humphrey gave her a
bronze hope chest as he proclaimed the space scientist the
National Multiple Sclerosis Society's Woman of the Year.

Her job often required travel to Cape Canaveral and Hous-
ton, and even an eclipse-tracking flight in a jetliner laboratory
eight miles above the earth. Lying on the floor of the plane to
focus on the sun's corona, she explained to the Mercury
astronaut with her what he should watch for on his flight
through space.

She confided to a close friend that before every flight she
would dehydrate herself because she knew she could never

reach a rest room aloft. With her total absorption in her work, she could take any inconvenience, accept any discomfort to keep going. By now, she was taking a daily rest on a couch in the NASA health unit and had to make the ultimate adjustment to her deteriorating condition. In January 1968 she discovered she could no longer walk from the elevator of her apartment building down the ramp to her car. Two men had to carry her and her crutches. After two days of that, she finally faced the full meaning of her physical limitations. She called the Multiple Sclerosis Society in Washington, and a wheelchair was delivered the same afternoon. When a battery-driven chair followed, she put the wheelchair trauma behind her and got back to business.

Her living arrangements became an increasing problem as she became unable to do anything for herself. Housekeepers ranged from bad to worse. On the other hand, her working arrangements enabled her to concentrate on the heavens with no earthly cares. NASA modified the doorways to the rest room on her floor so she could drive right in. A NASA nurse administered biweekly B-complex shots and accompanied her on out-of-town NASA business. A colleague drove her to work in exchange for the use of her "administrative parking permit." When her friend was not available, NASA provided someone to drive her. On Sundays, the minister himself drove her to church. A woman of pride as much as determination, she found difficulty in accepting the indignity of being unable even to bathe herself, but even greater difficulty in accepting retirement. When her director retired in 1973, she was urged to retire, too, to which she at first replied that she could not stop her mind and fifty-six was too young to retire. Then, she reflected, "I guess it's just as well. They're going to have a new regime, doing new things, not concerned so much with astronauts."

Multiple sclerosis may have shortened her career, but as a

friend commented: "She had nearly thirty good working years. How many people live to ninety and don't accomplish half what she did?"

Dr. Jocelyn Gill was able to surge ahead with her career because her disability worsened so slowly and because, by the time she needed help every inch of the way, she was so important to science in space that she got the help. With others, change comes faster or poses a more immediate threat to a career; they may have to alter their work plan—alter but not relinquish. Kathleen Shanahan Cohen had just completed medical school, pointing toward a career in obstetrics, when she had the first hint of a disease that would change her life. Two weeks after her internship began and the hospital ward was packed with polio cases, she suffered her first attack of double vision but still managed to do the spinal taps needed for positive diagnosis of polio. Through her years as an intern, attacks—cause still unnamed—periodically put her in the hospital as patient rather than doctor. She had already diagnosed her own illness before she was told what she had increasingly suspected. In those unenlightened days of the late 1940s, a diagnosis of multiple sclerosis was tantamount to a death sentence, or at least a vegetable existence, as the young doctor had seen on hospital wards.

"I had visions of this happening to me," she recalled. "The physical thing didn't bother me but I'd seen women in their twenties who didn't have their buttons." She put such thoughts from her mind but gave up the residency in obstetrics, which she knew would demand more time on her feet than she could manage. She could not give up medicine itself. Except for two months after the birth of her first child and four months after the second, she was never far from medicine. Writing about medicine rather than practicing it, she became assistant medical director of Pfizer International and editor of the drug company's journal. That gave her a chance to read every article that appeared on multiple sclerosis, even in French and German.

Dr. Shanahan Cohen was forty-one when she decided she had to come face to face with patients again. "I wanted to help people. Although I could justify medical writing, it wasn't that satisfying." At times, she could not walk four blocks without having to hold on to parking meters she passed, but she shrugged off physical limitations. She told her sister, Eileen, "I can be a shrink in a wheelchair as long as my head works." She took her residency in psychiatry at New York Medical College in 1962 and has been practicing ever since. For all the brave reference to a wheelchair life, she has been spared that step. The brace on her leg is hidden beneath a fashionable pants suit and she has turned her disability into an asset in treating patients. "Every doctor should be sick," she said. "I identify with my patients." Her being one of them helps her deal with their depressions.

The Multiple Sclerosis Society in Teaneck, New Jersey, where she practices, has an office in the same building and she volunteers to help her fellow victims. "I'm in the same boat as far as MS goes," she tells a man complaining about his wife. "There is no way you can look at yourself and not feel it's bloody unfair. You say what the hell did I do to deserve this. But nobody is out to get you. You know, it's not easy to live with somebody with MS."

The man heard her out, pondered her words, and then admitted, "You're right. My wife isn't being bitchy like I said. She just runs out of patience."

Recalling the exchange, the psychiatrist said the man had apparently given up but now decided to train as a real estate salesman. He stopped sulking at home and feeling sorry for himself because, as he told Dr. Shanahan Cohen, "You get into the office every day, so why should I feel sorry for myself?"

She gets into more than one office. She is clinical assistant

professor of psychiatry at the New Jersey College of Medicine
and Dentistry in Newark, consulting psychiatrist for the
Bergen Community College in Paramus, and in the private
practice of psychiatry, child psychiatry, and psychoanalysis.
She has been much involved in medical women's associations,
Democratic politics, and her temple, and, at one time, was a
member of the local board of education. "I find something challenging every day of the week," she says. Probably that was
why she was named 1977 Woman of the Year by the New
Jersey Medical Women's Association.

What keeps her going, she says, is "the sense that you have
some real meaning to people and they do to you." She is sus-
tained by the knowledge that she is "a functioning person who
is useful to this world."

The most disabled man I know, the one who can move nothing but his head, filled six important posts until a heart attack
in 1977. Now he contents himself with five of them. Multiple
sclerosis has wholly crippled his body, but his spirit remains
undimmed.

Dr. Joseph J. Panzarella, Jr., the 1977 Handicapped American of the Year, has had more than enough trials and torments
to defeat a lesser man. During World War II, he completed
medical school in uniform. He was twenty-five years old when
a slight limp and a weakness in one arm led to a diagnosis of
multiple sclerosis and his discharge from the army.

He told his longtime sweetheart that he might be disabled
and not able to practice medicine, but she paid no attention.
That was the most fortunate thing that ever happened to him.
They were married a week before he got his medical degree.
Jo's constant loving presence has made his spectacular career
possible.

On bad advice, he went into anesthesiology, which he found
very grueling, though he asked no quarter. One icy morning
in 1952, a car plowed into him. He could no longer work as

well, nor do anesthetics—a doctor said he might have injured his spinal cord. An operation left him more crippled and very depressed.

More than a year of staying home ended suddenly when Jo Panzarella's pregnancy with twins—the seventh and eighth child in ten years—went sour. Her husband insisted on going to the hospital to be with her. He managed to get his wheelchair up to the car, crawled in, put a foot on the gas and a foot on the brake, and drove for the first time since his damaging operation. The twins died, but the doctor and his wife were together.

When he started job hunting in medicine, prospective employers raised objections to hiring a wheelchair-bound doctor —an experience he has never forgotten. He has, therefore, become the champion of the disabled. "I feel if I can show that I can do it, the nondisabled would be more amenable to giving opportunity to others."

Dr. Howard A. Rusk, head of the Institute of Rehabilitation Medicine and pioneer in the field, gave him that opportunity. With a Rusk fellowship, he trained at the institute. The day he finished, he had a job there. He was still able to drive and push his wheelchair around. As he progressed to complete paralysis he moved up in his chosen field. He became director of the Chronic Care, Physical Medicine, and Rehabilitation Center in the Brunswick Hospital Center at Amityville, Long Island; director of the department of rehabilitation medicine at Franklin General Hospital, Valley Stream; professor of physical therapy and other subjects at the New York University Post-Graduate Medical School; member of the faculty of Nassau Community College and Suffolk Community College on Long Island; and rehabilitation consultant for the Continental Insurance Company—a New York City job he reluctantly gave up after a heart attack.

An earlier heart attack tested him as nothing before. His

son Jeff, with whom he was very close, had helped him into the ambulance and told him, "I'll take you out of it at the hospital." But Jeff was not there to take him out and it fell to Jo to keep her husband from knowing that their son had hit a telephone pole and died on his way to the hospital to help his father. She kept up the fiction for three days by staggering the visits of their children, but when one of them came for the second time, Dr. Panzarella knew something had happened to Jeff.

The doctor was hit hard again a few years ago when he noticed his daughter Jackie limping, her symptoms a replica of his own. Jackie was the tomboy of the family, the one who climbed fences, the cheerleader. Tests confirmed what he had suspected. Jackie said, "If daddy can do it, can make of his life what he has, I can make it." And she has. She accomplished what she wanted most—a baby.

Dr. Panzarella lives what he preaches. He knows his physical limitations but also his mental strengths. "I know I can't walk, but I can have someone push my chair. As long as I can use my mind, I can function. The body is just the vehicle for the mind."

One of his patients agreed: "He may not be able to move his body, but he sure can move his mind."

He devised methods to budget his time and adapt his duties so he can perform them. A mechanical lift moves him from car to wheelchair. He dictates to a staff of secretaries via a telephone intercom recording system. Patients are positioned so he can look them in the eye and converse easily. A nurse holds his stethoscope and other instruments.

"I know what I can do," Dr. Panzarella said. "I've made peace with myself. I live within my abilities. It's my way of life. I feel that being able to do that, I'm contributing to others who are disabled and who need an example."

Some of my other new friends have had to give up what

they were doing, what they were trained to do, but for them, too, the disease seems to act as a spur to bring out this need to be of some use to others as well as themselves.

At thirty-six, Robert D. Douglas had to relinquish his career as a virologist at the National Institutes of Health when an attack of multiple sclerosis left him with a feeling of total exhaustion and inability to concentrate. He had tremors in his hands, loss of vision, and assaults of great pain. Yet he regards his multiple sclerosis as a blessing in disguise because it made him aware of the needs of handicapped children and gave him an unbelievably effective way to help them.

The first symptoms had appeared nearly a decade earlier when dizziness and loss of peripheral vision put him in the hospital. A spinal tap revealed nothing and he went back to work. In 1971, the symptoms returned, this time in much worse form. One leg became crippled. After hospital tests, he was told he had a demyelinating disease. He knew what that meant because he was then studying viruses that cause demyelination. He knew multiple sclerosis was a demyelinating disease, although it still is unproven that a virus causes it. He was familiar with the symptoms but refused to believe they fitted him. Less than a year later, when he experienced total loss of his eyesight, total loss of the use of his left leg, and partial loss of strength in his right arm, he went to Johns Hopkins University Hospital, where doctors diagnosed his case as multiple sclerosis.

He knew he would have to give up his study of viruses at the National Institutes of Health, because "I wasn't seeing things too clearly. I could mess up an experiment." But he realized that if he did not work he would have too much time to think about himself. He had explained to his wife of nearly twenty years and his two daughters, now twelve and sixteen, exactly what multiple sclerosis did to the body and could do.

Now he called a family conference to discuss work they could all do together.

Douglas had been riding for fifteen years before the onset of multiple sclerosis. He had kept a horse at a stable under a National Park Service concession in Washington's Rock Creek Park. The stable was up for sale and he and his wife bought it with a partner, whom they bought out in a year.

Despite the demands of an eighty-horse stable, despite frequent twelve-hour days, despite an almost unbearable pain in his legs, he took on another career. It began when a little girl with cerebral palsy came out to see the horses. She had no control of her legs, her muscle tone was gone, and she was frothing at the mouth because she had no control over her glands. She was wearing a helmet to protect her when she fell. She begged to get on a horse. Could she ride a pony? her teacher asked. Douglas got her mother's hesitant permission and put the six-year-old in the saddle. That was in August 1972. By February, 1973, she was riding twice a week, her grades in school had improved, and she needed her helmet only when riding. Convinced that horseback riding could help other handicapped children, Douglas called the school board and offered to teach free if somebody would get the children to the stable. He began with ten emotionally disturbed youngsters, ten physically handicapped, and ten mentally retarded. The results were so fantastic that the school system set up a budget and made horseback riding part of the curriculum for handicapped children. Douglas's wife, Dorothy, took a year off from teaching to develop a classroom guide to reinforce what the children learned at the stable. Instead of reading about Dick and Jane, the children read about horses. The value of the therapy went far beyond ease of their suffering and unearthed their buried instinct for play. By learning to groom the horses, rub them down, feed and water them, braid their tails and manes, they found self-confidence and self-esteem in a world that had shunned or pitied them.

Douglas said, "They have come to understand some things about themselves and others."

When you see a blind girl, with her blond hair tucked into a hunting cap, jump a fence on her mare, you begin to believe anything is possible there. "Take the children who come out here in wheelchairs," Douglas pointed out as we strolled around the stable. "Can you imagine the psychological boost for a child who can't walk and then suddenly is riding on four legs through Rock Creek Park?"

The psychological boost is not limited to the children. Douglas admits he would have given up the horse center as too much work if it were not for the four hundred children he serves now. They come from twelve schools—deaf children with a riding instructor who talks to them in sign language, retarded and emotionally disturbed children, ones who have trouble learning, and others who cannot walk or cannot see. Douglas does not discriminate against any of them, no matter how handicapped.

When he was healthy, swimming miles, jogging, and playing squash, Douglas never thought about the handicapped. Now he thinks of nothing but the children he sees growing and changing. "When I see a boy who has been in a wheelchair all his life being able to control his body enough to get on a horse and walk through the park, that is my reward."

The stable stays busy with healthy as well as handicapped riders and teaching can be a full-time job, but employees at the center very seldom say to him, "Let me do that for you" or, "Why don't you go in and rest?" They know he wants no sympathy; when he is ready to go in and rest, he will. "They treat me as any normal person will treat another normal person."

The stable has brought his family closer together. The girls have become excellent riders and his wife visits the stable frequently. He sees his family more now than he did when he was working on his old eight-hour job.

"I used to try to project what I would be doing a year from now or five years from now, but what I project now is today. If I can make it through today, then today is complete, and tomorrow I'll start a new day. Sometimes it is a curse, sometimes a blessing. Because of the children I can help, I find it a blessing more often than a curse."

The achievers with multiple sclerosis have much in common besides the disease that has forced their lives in new directions. Characteristically, they refuse to feel sorry for themselves or to accept pity. Their work is enhanced by a new sensitivity to the distress of others. And they have come to terms with their disease. They may even use it to get more out of life, as Robert Douglas has done, as Gary Smith, a mountain eagle with clipped wings, is trying to do.

In 1975, before multiple sclerosis struck, Smith was known in the mountain West as a modern renaissance man—a strapping, six-foot-four, two-hundred-pound athlete who quoted poetry, a ranger who composed songs about man's debt to nature, an author who celebrated the simple folk in lyric prose, a guitar-strumming folk singer, and a fierce environmentalist. As a marine stationed on Okinawa, he would run nine miles a day just for the fun of it. In his beloved mountains, he would climb three Tetons in one day. He had been a ranger in Canyonlands National Park and, before that, the first U.S. Forest Service naturalist and wilderness patrolman on the rugged Sawtooth Mountain of Idaho.

While he was a back-country ranger he had a rafting accident on the Colorado River. Shortly afterward, he felt an electric buzzing sensation in his spine. The buzzing continued as he worked on the early stages of writing and assembling *Windsinger,* his somewhat autobiographical environmental odyssey. In March 1975 a major attack left him temporarily unable to focus his eyes or keep his balance. He would wake up with his fingers too numb to strum his guitar and "catch" his tunes. His book was delayed when he could no longer focus on the words he had written. He had to give up flying because his eyes could no longer be trusted to bring him safely home.

"Flying offers such a fantastic overview," he recalled. "Life is seeing the whole picture and connecting it all up. You can do that with a piece of wild land from the air. Maybe this enforced limitation will cause me to look closer at what's right here—the rock on the table or the texture of those leaves—things similar in a way to the people in my book—maybe noticed, but not seen." Although he may talk like a philosopher, Gary is no sedentary graybeard. His beard is dark brown, as much a part of his look of the mountain West as his fringed jacket and boots, and he is rarely sedentary.

He will say, in a burst of introspection, "I've always listened to nature and she's never done me wrong. And I think perhaps my sickness is nature's way of telling me to turn inward now to finish the task she has given me." To Smith, the task is to save our natural resources for future generations. To him, that means fighting the encroachment of power plants in western wild lands, demanding a massive effort to alter the country's energy technology, railing against what is being done to plunder our planet. So he blithely writes to the president of the United States and family. He wants the president to declare an energy war, defining the enemy and the nation's mission but providing the tools to do the job. He prays "that any national gear-changing would be guided by a commitment to respect the rights of all creatures in the ecosystem so we will be successful in passing a healthier earth on to our children."

In the heat of a southwestern summer he lived in a pueblo and worked in the fields to learn how the Indians lived, how they become so intuitive that they know what you are going to ask before you know yourself. The heat hit him, as it will do with multiple sclerosis. He went blind.

Six weeks later, his eyesight returned and he was at it again, scrambling over rocks, taking over the controls of an airplane to get it in a better position to make spectacular photographs, hiking and jeeping into the most rugged and remote areas. He took a jeep over country so rough that it took seven and a half hours to go forty-six miles. He was seeking primitive art on the rocks of the wilderness and on the walls of caves. "The earth was their canvas," he said. "Their art is as great as Picasso and helps offset our arrogance as a people."

"Yes," I interrupted, "but how do you feel?"

"The legs are okay," he said, "except that the right leg has been acting funny, probably by the way I was sitting in the jeep. But I've been very strong. The other day, I did a ten-mile hike with fifty pounds of equipment in the moonlight through the snow."

Then he was back to talking about his wilderness find. "The art on the rocks are a lot of road signs of time. We found only one modern sign, the only one in English. Carved on a rock were the words, 'Man first landed on moon.' "

His enthusiasm touches everything he does, every person he meets. One girl is hardly likely to forget a note he had left on her car: "Remember we exist only to discover beauty. All else is a form of waiting." With his book now in its second printing and scheduled to come out in paperback, with a record of his songs to complement the book, with an honorable mention for investigative reporting to crow about, with several magazine articles in the works, he simply cannot afford to let multiple sclerosis become more than a minor inconvenience. "I've got a lot to say to people," he says, "and a lot to share. I'm the kind of person who has never taken life for granted. I could lose it all tomorrow and I wouldn't feel cheated. Every day for me is a bonus."

And he resumes strumming his guitar as he changes the illustrations of his songs by shifting the slides with his big toe. My friends and many others like them refuse to retreat. They simply redesign their lives—after they go through the same anguished, soul-searching "why me?" as everyone else.

Tony Rodolakis, the research physicist who had shifted from a think-tank job to a new career as a stockbroker just before multiple sclerosis struck, was forced to rest evenings instead of going out on the town like the carefree bachelor of old. Lying on his bed for hours at a time, he developed mathematical theories about the stock market. He wrote a book about it, *Buying Options: Wall Street on a Shoestring.* The enforced rest is now paying off in book sales.

Jacqueline du Pre has not wholly forsaken her beloved cello. Now thirty-two, she has been in a wheelchair since her spectacular international career was cut short. Now she can coax sound only with difficulty from the Stradivarius cello given her by an unknown admirer, but friends who have heard her play in private say she can still produce beauty of sound despite wrong notes. The soaring tones of a cello still sound from Jacqueline du Pre's London home, but someone else is playing—one of the advanced pupils who come to her for her interpretation of the music. She considers herself lucky because she has been able to alter the direction of her artistic energy into teaching. It was lucky, too, she says, that her musical ability was discovered early and that she had progressed quickly to performances so that when her career ended at twenty-eight she had already won the plaudits of the world and lived a richly rewarding artistic life.

You don't have to be a star, or at the top of your profession, to move with grace and even eagerness into a new life-style. For one woman the disease made a dream attainable. She had been a teacher for fourteen years, wanting to write, never finding time or energy. After she was stricken, her husband bought a farm in Pennsylvania. He farms, she writes, and they are living their dream life.

One man had devoted his working life to building a business in surplus military goods. When the disease made a full day at the store no longer possible, he sold the business to his son. Now father works for son, but also finds time to pass along his fund of business know-how to young people with the disease. Another man, nearing sixty, had to give up his government job. He kept his political interests, his girl friend, and his sailing club, and stays busy with a small mail order business in office supplies—including his own invention: a filing device.

Morton Jaffe and his wife have been working together in an accounting firm for the past fifteen or twenty years. Half that time, he has had multiple sclerosis and now goes to work in a wheelchair, but he goes—five days a week from 7:30 A.M. to 4:30 P.M. "I'm getting stronger all the time," Jaffe insists. He believes his determination is a matter of his physical makeup. "It's what's inside you. If you're a fighter, you fight, you don't give in."

But suppose you gave up a job because it was too much for you only to find now you are in remission or your miseries are under control? Or suppose disease struck before you had a chance to test yourself on your first job? Many of you need training or retraining before you can enter or reenter the job market. Many of you hesitate because you think employers will turn away from a girl who walks with a limp or a man in a wheelchair. Thousands of potential employers all over the country do not dare turn away from the disabled anymore. It could cost them lucrative government contracts. That is government policy, a policy now being enforced.

It is likewise government policy to help the handicapped stay on the jobs they have by changing their work environment to meet their changed physical condition. Multiple sclerosis damaged a friend's eyes, but his job, which required much telephoning, was saved when his telephone dial was fitted with enlarged numbers. Another friend was ready to quit because driving to work had become too much for his weakened legs. Hand controls on his automobile have kept him in business. Those were routine assists from a local department of vocational rehabilitation. It is far easier for the employer to adjust a job to fit the handicap than for the disabled employee to start job hunting all over again.

Whether a person with multiple sclerosis is trying to stay on the job or get on the job, any local department of vocational rehabilitation should now be ready to help. Late in 1977, the National Multiple Sclerosis Society, HEW's Rehabilitation Services Administration, and the Council of State Administrators of Vocational Rehabilitation joined in a statement of "principles of cooperation." The target set in the agreement was for state vocational rehabilitation agencies to work with ten thousand multiple sclerosis patients annually, graduating about twenty-five hundred into the work force each year, instead of the six hundred to seven hundred in state programs at the time of the agreement. Some $20 million is expected to be spent annually.

Counselors help the handicapped worker develop a work goal and provide necessary aids—whether it be training for a new skill, a wheelchair to get the training, or equipment needed to stay on the old job. An agency bought one girl an electric typewriter because she was studying for a degree to reach her work goal and needed to type her examination papers. Her standard typewriter was no longer usable because she could not hit the keys hard enough. The soft touch of the electric typewriter was all she could manage.

Under a more enlightened interpretation of the law, homemaking is considered an employment goal, too. That is particularly meaningful for women with multiple sclerosis trying desperately to keep their homes going and their families happy. A handicapped homemaker can now get a swivel stool to park in front of her kitchen counter. Enthroned on the stool, she can swing one way to reach the silverware and another to get the salad fixings from the refrigerator. She can reign again over her kitchen.

People with multiple sclerosis have long been as handicapped by prejudices of prospective employers as by the disease itself. That picture is changing, partially by the more open attitude of people with the disease but even more by government action.

Under a federal law passed in the early 1970s, contractors and subcontractors holding contracts with the United States must take "affirmative action" to ensure equal employment opportunity for all qualified workers. That means the thirty thousand or more contractors selling goods and services to the government, and even more subcontractors with contracts for more than $2,500, are supposed to do more than simply hire those who apply and promote them without discrimination. They are also expected to go out looking for qualified women, minority workers, the handicapped, and veterans. Further, they are supposed to make a "reasonable" effort to accommodate the special needs of the handicapped. Thus, they cannot refuse to hire someone because a wheelchair will not fit under the desk. They are supposed to raise the desk.

The way things worked out, though, women and minority workers got attention earlier than the handicapped and veterans (often the same thing). Until late 1977, the Department of Labor's Office of Federal Contract Compliance Programs took no action against employers discriminating against handicapped and veterans unless they filed individual complaints that a federal contractor or subcontractor refused them jobs for which they were qualified or passed over them for promotion or fired them solely because of their handicap. When a complaint was filed, the compliance office in Washington, or one of the ten regional offices, would investigate and try to resolve the dispute. As of the end of 1977, 120 people across the country had received some $360,000 in back pay. The first step toward strengthening the antidiscrimination program for the handicapped and veterans—the two short-changed groups in the drive for equal employment opportunity —came in late 1977 when the government began to bring formal charges against companies accused of discriminating against the handicapped because they were handicapped. The penalty could be loss of a federal contract, often by far the most lucrative part of a company's business. By early 1978, the government had brought charges against five companies, some of them leaders of their industries. They are not taken into court—the action is called an administrative complaint— but it could take them out of their government contracts.

Early in 1978, the Department of Labor began putting the handicapped and veterans on a par with women and minorities. Ever since equal employment opportunity became a legal right, investigators had been reviewing industries to find pockets of prejudice against women and minorities. Investigators would select prime contractors at random or by industry or the size of a contract; study pay records; dig deep into the professional attitudes of middle- and high-level management; interview personnel people, always looking for deeply ingrained antipathy against a particular group. Now industries and individual employers with government contracts also will be canvassed to make sure they are actively trying to put qualified but handicapped people and veterans on their payrolls, too, and give them an opportunity to rise to the positions their talents merit.

Until recently, I would tell handicapped friends to try for a government job because I knew government agencies are continually alerting staffs to hire the handicapped, to welcome them to their ranks. Now, I say, "Try for a job with an outfit that holds a government contract for more than $2,500." And that covers an unbelievably wide range. It could be a job with an airline. Most airlines have government contracts to haul personnel and packages. It could be a company supplying beef to bears at a federal zoo. From A to Z, the government is in everything, and a handicapped person could be, too. Don't expect the same clout yet in companies dealing with state and local governments because the federal government's quickened interest in helping the handicapped to help themselves is just beginning to filter down to city and state governments.

Some companies are reaching for new ways to make working life not only possible but comfortable for the disabled. Typical of them is an IBM installation in Gaithersburg, Maryland, where seven multiple sclerosis victims work. There, a security guard at the door helps disabled employees out of their cars with their wheelchairs and gets them into the building. Sometimes, when the disabled want to use a wheelchair only to reach a distant office, a security guard locks up the wheelchair overnight near the entrance, where it will be available for the long trek the next morning.

In some offices, fellow workers band together to make sure their friend with multiple sclerosis will be able to continue working beside them. A woman at the Federal Bureau of Investigation knows that on days when she lacks the strength to drive herself to work, one of several people in her office will pick her up. At lunchtime, one of them keeps a place for her in the long cafeteria line to spare her legs the toll of a long wait. Another friend finds a table near the cafeteria check-out so she will have a shorter distance to walk.

For the person with multiple sclerosis, whether long in remission or just recovering from an attack, the chances today of getting and holding a job are better than they have ever been. If they can possibly manage it, they are far better off working full time because they will have less opportunity to feel sorry for themselves, more opportunity to pride themselves on their accomplishments. Others have climbed the job ladder with a gimpy leg. They can, too.

Chapter 6

Coping

Barbara McGrath goes to market every two weeks, leaving it to her husband to pick up milk and eggs between her shopping excursions. Clutching her ten-cents-off coupons and her list of today's specials, she wheels into the supermarket and stakes out a shopping cart. She leaves the cart at the end of an aisle and begins to wheel herself up one aisle and down another, piling groceries on her lap.

When her lap is full, she wheels back to her staked-out shopping cart and unloads. To make her unloading trips shorter, she gives the cart a little shove to get it a few aisles further along. When the day's marketing is done, her husband and boys bring her haul into the house but she puts the groceries away herself because she wants to know where everything is.

As Barbara knows better than most, our most treasured possession is our independence, our self-reliance, our ability to think for ourselves and do for ourselves.

We face barriers, however, that we never dreamed existed. Stepping up a curb can become a major hazard. Even holding a book may require help. Unexpected physical limitations confront us as we see functions lost and not always regained, living arrangements that must be altered, daily chores requiring an imagination we never thought we had.

Learning to cope with our new life can be a full-time job until we discover the dos and don'ts of our condition. At the same time, though, we may discover that if one has to be disabled, it could not come at a better time. The disabled used to be handicapped from taking their place in the mainstream not only by injury or disease but by too narrow doorways and other architectural barriers. They are now, however, the newest favored minority with many champions to plead their cause. Any discrimination against them becomes a major civil rights issue. The wheelchair brigade has become a force in our society to be reckoned with and cheered.

Distinctions between the able and disabled are narrowing every day as new state and federal laws ensure that architectural barriers come down in public facilities from subways to swimming pools, from state and city universities to national parks. Still, change does not come overnight, since alterations to give access to the handicapped apply primarily to new facilities, and governments hate to spend money until they have to. Nevertheless, the changes *are* coming, and it is up to us to make full use of them.

Many of the tricks and tips, the dos and don'ts for multiple sclerosis that follow, apply to any person with any disability. This is a cookbook of coping recipes in alphabetical order.

BACKACHE: With our spine out of alignment and our walk throwing us off balance, backaches follow. A heating pad might ease the pain but concentrated heat weakens us. A massage will help if someone is around to do the massaging. Swimming might get out the kinks but a swimming pool is not always available. Usually, a pain killer is too drastic a solution for an ache that can be better helped by exercise. (See chapter 7.)

BATH AND TOILET: Bathing poses special problems for those who cannot stand in a shower and who have trouble climbing in and out of a tub. These measures help: a bathtub safety rail secured to the side of the tub, grab bars on the wall, tub seat and tub transfer board to slide from wheelchair to seat, settling for a sponge bath on bad days, putting a chair in the shower stall to enjoy a pulsating hand-held shower. Other useful bathroom equipment: an easily removed raised toilet seat for patients with weak or stiffened legs, a floating thermometer for those who cannot feel whether water is hot or cold, a bathbrush with an 180-degree curved handle to help those with limited range of motion scrub back and shoulders, a toothbrush with a built-up foam rubber handle, a long-handled toothpaste tube squeezer.

BLADDER AND BOWEL PROBLEMS: Incontinence can be the most important problem, making some patients depressed, withdrawn, reluctant to travel, difficult to live with, less confident at work. Others cover their embarrassment with laughter and candidly tell associates the meeting will have to break for what they call a "potty stop." To avoid bladder problems and a possibly dangerous infection, a nurse-victim suggests emptying the bladder every two hours and drinking five quarts of fluid daily, including cranberry juice to maintain urine acidity. Another nurse, a patient herself, favors keeping a two-week record of the time, amount, and kind of fluid drunk and the number of times and amount voided. Then, she says, habits can be evaluated and altered. She limits fluids herself before going out, takes only one drink at parties, and locates the bathroom and its light switch before drinking at all. At a meeting or show, she always visits the rest room before taking her seat. Accidents are minor and infrequent and can be minimized by cutting a diaper in four parts to wear. Men can solve the problem with a bladder bag. Drugs can be helpful, if the doctor approves, and so can exercise. (See chapter 7.)

Learn to recognize symptoms of urinary infection and call your doctor at the first sign of trouble. Never postpone treatment because you fear a bladder problem may mean lifelong catheterization. That may never happen because physicians are increasingly able to manage bladder problems with intermittent catheterization, medication, and other new techniques.

While the bowel misbehaves less frequently than the bladder, when it does it can have disastrous effects. Unless one wants always to wear Pampers, anybody prone to bowel problems should avoid laxatives when planning to go out and should get to the bathroom at the first indication of a bowel explosion. One should never delay to read another page or finish a conversation. It will not wait.

BOREDOM: Having too little to occupy you can make you more tired than a full day at the office used to do. You start feeling sorry for yourself and that launches the downhill slide. One woman told me when she gets out early in the morning, even in her wheelchair, she can stick with a project well into afternoon, but if she stays home she is ready for bed by lunchtime.

To avoid the weakening effects of idleness, you might consider a part-time job when you can no longer work full time. (See chapter 5.) If you have trouble getting around, consider working at home but only for a person or agency you know. If you have to pay out even a dollar to start working at home, check first with your Better Business Bureau or Postal Inspection Service. Your Multiple Sclerosis Society can always use your help on a research project or to provide telephone reassurance to those who have recently discovered their illness. You can also join a group meeting periodically for discussion of everything from problems of the disease to flower-arranging or Oriental cooking. You can go into politics by helping a candidate rally votes. You can develop a new interest, preferably one that makes money or helps others. You will reap your greatest dividend in the new friends you make, and that is something we never needed more.

CANES: For more than a year, I used an umbrella instead of a cane, even on sunny days. When people asked me if I expected rain, I said I carried the umbrella to make sure of sunshine and they should thank me for it. Now that I use a cane, I realize how stupid I was. One winter day, I reached a curb to find a sheet of ice in my path, much too wide for me to step across. Helplessly, I leaned on my cane and glanced around. A chivalrous man stepped up to help me across the ice patch and another got me to the curb on the other side. The cane had signaled my need.

A cane also saves explanations when a walk becomes a stagger. A girl I know who was having a bad day used her hand on the wall to steady herself as she made her way back to her office. The office kidder, noticing her unsteady progress, asked, "What kind of a liquid lunch did *you* have today?" She told him she had multiple sclerosis and watched his embarrassed flush, but the incident could have been avoided if she had carried a cane. A friend considers his an explanation-saver. He uses the cane when he goes out on dates to establish quickly that he has multiple sclerosis, that if the room heats up he must leave, and that he may have to excuse himself to go to the men's room several times during the evening. With that behind them, no other explanations are necessary. When strangers ask him why a young man like him uses a cane—as strangers do to all cane-users—he replies briskly: "I use it to fight off pretty girls and beat up old ladies and kids with dirty faces!"

Carrying a cane saves falls and enables us to go farther afield. We are inclined to venture forth without realizing that our legs may start to drag before we are halfway home, although we feel fine now. With a cane, we can make it all the way. A cane does not have to look like something out of a hospital supply room. It can be a silver-headed ebony cane or have a conversation-piece handle that even the able-bodied admire. For parties and travel, I use a cane that folds into four sections. The instant I pull it from its case, it straightens automatically. I can keep it folded and inconspicuous until I really need it, and when I pull it out, I can make a show of it, like Merlin the Magician.

CLOTHING: Today's loose and layered look for women and casual men's fashions make dressing much easier for people who cannot tie a shoelace or tie, cannot button a blouse or shirt, and may not be able to lift their arms enough to put on a hat. You can slip into loafers, using a shoehorn if necessary, instead of tying laces. An ascot or turtleneck sweater, instead of a tie, is all the fashion. Hats are seldom worn even in winter. On a cold day, a woman can toss a wool scarf over the head, tucked into the coat without needing to be tied. Women who prefer blouses to sweaters choose zippers and front fasteners instead of buttons. A gadget on a long chain can hook into your zipper to pull it up for you when you cannot reach around back to do it yourself. Snap-on fasteners, easy for numb fingers to manage, are showing up in more and more clothing. If you are still stuck with buttons, a buttoner with a wire loop circles the button so it can be pulled through the hole.

Today's fashions divert attention from our problems and toward our attractions. Decorated vests bring the eye above the waist rather than down to stiff legs. Women who need braces on their legs can conceal them beneath pants suits by day and long dresses or caftans by night. Elasticized waist-bands make belt buckling unnecessary. Loose sleeves replace ones that end with buttoned cuffs. Fashionable boots tend to keep the foot in one position, preventing turned ankles and tripping. Finally, the current full-skirted evening gowns make a woman look feminine, attractive, and very much "with it" even in a wheelchair.

COLDS: We have to be more careful than healthy people to ward off colds because a cough accompanied by fever may trigger an attack. Make a point of keeping away from people with the flu or a cold, and if you must kiss, do so only out of real affection, not just to say hello. My method is always to turn the other cheek. During flu season, stay off crowded buses and out of movie houses. Your television programs may not be X-rated but you should not be heated up anyway, and staying home is one way to escape bugs.

COOKING: Your best friend is your freezer. Since you can no longer run to the store every day, you have to buy for a week or more at a time and store it. One woman alone buys for a month, cooks, and freezes her meals in bags. Another, who cooks from a wheelchair, waits for a "good day," and prepares several dishes for her family of four. She will cook a large dish of lasagna and freeze what remains. She says her children like it better the second time—something about the juices. She can prepare a turkey dinner from her wheelchair, but when the turkey weight is above twelve pounds, she gets it ready and waits for her husband to put it in the oven. Her wheelchair gives her mobility to get around her kitchen. When she has all her supplies together on her lap, she puts them on the counter and shifts to a high-backed stool to prepare the meal. When she entertains, she wheels the dishes to the buffet and everyone serves himself.

Burns and scalds are a constant hazard for fingers that lose their grip and arms that lose coordination. Long asbestos-fabric oven mitts can prevent painful and unsightly burns. Pots with handles and covers can prevent burning liquid from slopping over when the pots are lifted. Rather than spilling soup enroute to the table, I put empty plates at the table and pour the soup just before the guests sit down to dinner.

DEPRESSION: For most of us, depression is a passing phase when we confront something we used to do but can do no more. Here are ways some of my friends haul themselves out of depression:

A former super-salesman: "I use exactly the same techniques I used selling. Part of it is physical—to screw a smile on your face and say something happy. Part is mental—to give yourself a boot in the tail and get out of it."

A former golf champion: "I pick up my knitting, turn on television, and think of others worse off than me, like the woman I saw at the MS dinner who couldn't even feed herself."

A secretary: "I have a good cry and go to sleep, and in the morning I'm fine."

A psychiatrist: "When I'm down, I say let's see what happens tomorrow and something good happens and the depression disappears."

Some others, including me, try to create something to push away unwanted thoughts. When I am angry or sad or depressed, I take it out on the typewriter.

DIET, VITAMINS, AND "CURES": Victims fall regularly for what one friend calls the "peanut butter syndrome." "If somebody eats peanut butter and it coincides with an upcycle in his disease, he's going to say peanut butter is a cure for MS. People don't say they stopped eating peanut butter because they ate it when they went down. It's always the ups they talk about." That may sound far-fetched but so are some diet theories, vitamin fantasies, and "sure cures."

One man visited me with a suitcase full of vitamins—a day's supply. A friend told me he used to spend forty-five minutes every morning just putting vitamin pills in bottles. "At the rate I was popping pills when I decided to stop my mega-vitamin therapy, my fix was costing me $40 a week." Another friend said he spent thousands of dollars and every Sunday night sorting out the fifty he had to take at each meal until he, too, quit. A doctor concluded that with an adequate diet, there is no need to take vitamin pills that you shove in one end and out the other.

As for "cures," the National Multiple Sclerosis Society periodically announces it is supporting research to determine the value, if any, of various curative drugs and devices, but so far has found nothing to support the claims of inventors or the dreams of victims. The society always advises patients to listen to their own physicians.

Over the past three decades, many diets—some conflicting with each other—have won followers but no scientific study yet conclusively finds any relationship between diet and multiple sclerosis. The National Multiple Sclerosis Society takes the position that until it gets scientific proof that any diet can alter the course of multiple sclerosis, a well-balanced, richly varied diet with all the needed food elements recommended by scientific nutritionists is the way to go. As a guide to a healthy diet within the framework of the disease, the society recently issued a booklet entitled *Nutrition and MS* by Dr. Simmons, the society's former director of medical programs.

Dr. Helmut J. Bauer of West Germany, international authority on multiple sclerosis, states flatly that a diet capable of healing multiple sclerosis does not exist. He suggests a diet framework of sensible nutrition, a limited amount of fats with a high proportion of polyunsaturated fatty acids, and a low-cholesterol intake, a liberal amount of animal and plant protein, liberal amounts of preferably fresh fruits and vegetables, a limited sugar intake and a preference for cereals, rice, grain products, and potatoes, avoiding gravies and fried food. A daily intake of 1,800 calories can be maintained with tasty and varied foods and yes, you can dress up your dishes with spices (and a moderate amount of salt), despite a widespread idea that spices should be prohibited for multiple sclerosis patients.

DRINKING: Friends do people with multiple sclerosis no favor when they urge them to take another drink. If nothing else, alcohol worsens an already shaky coordination and makes it more difficult to walk, talk, type, play the piano, or concentrate. When a nervous system is already damaged, alcohol may be the one assault too many. If you are going to have a drink, do it at home, where you know the way not only to the bathroom but to bed.

DRIVING: With hand controls, people whose legs fail them still can drive. A man who had been housebound for a year, reluctant to ask others to drive him, discovered hand controls and promptly tooled around the neighborhood. "Hey," he shouted to passing friends, "my wife doesn't even know where I am. Isn't that great!" Any Department of Vocational Rehabilitation will pay for hand controls that make possible a return to work.

Special license plates with the wheelchair symbol on them or, in some states, an H.P. (for "handicapped person") enable motorists with walking problems to park in reserved spaces near building entrances. These parking places are usually wider than normal to allow for passage of a wheelchair.

The car itself can become an aid. One man I know stores

the parts of his Amigo in the rear of his station wagon and
then works his way to the driver's seat by grasping the luggage
rack atop his wagon.

EATING: If you are eating out, choose a restaurant with a
rest room on the same floor. If you have trouble cutting your
meat, your waiter can serve it already cut. At home, many
gadgets—some of which you can devise yourself—make eating easier. If you cannot hold a glass or straw, get a card-
board lid to fit over the glass, punch a hole in the lid and
stick in a straw. Weighted knives and forks keep food from
flying around, and handles can be built up with a wrapping
of foam rubber for hands with a weak grasp. Partitioned
dishes can keep food from spilling on the table. A number of
self-help aids to eating are now available by mail.*

EMOTIONS AND STRESS: One night an old friend called to
ask if I would like to see the new James Bond movie. The
unexpected excursion made me as happy as a first date. The
next day four people told me I was walking better than I had
in a long time. They were so emphatic about it that I checked
it out with a psychologist. Could a happy feeling have that
much physical effect? "Absolutely," she replied. "Emotions
play an extremely important part in this whole illness. Patients have told me that when they feel depressed, feel anxious,
or have a fight with someone, they fall a lot more and don't
walk as well. When they feel contented, feel good about themselves, they do much better." She said my experience was
typical.

Any stressful situation immediately backfires in physical
problems. I saw a girl walking quite normally, even striding,
before she learned she was to go to a job interview that after-

* Fred Sammons, Inc.; *BeOK* self-help aids; Professional and Institutional
Catalogue for 1978; Toll-free Order Phone—800/323-7305, Illinois calls—
312/971-0610; or Order by Mail—Box 32, Brookfield, Illinois 60513.

noon. The prospect of the interview bothered her so much that by lunchtime she was lurching instead of walking and her usually clipped speech had become slurred.

My friends try to avoid upsets and arguments by dealing with disputes when they can manage them best. One mother tells her teen-agers that she is not at her best at the end of the day so that is no time to ask for permission to do some things. They will fare better in the morning. She tries to avoid end-of-day skirmishes with her husband. If he starts waving bills at her then, she will say, "See you later. I'm going to watch TV." Usually, he understands.

ENJOYING LIFE: You can moon over times past and opportunities lost, an attitude guaranteed to get you down. Or you can make whatever adjustments you need to keep on having fun and appreciate the simple pleasures you were too busy to notice before. Some of my bicycling friends now ride tandem with healthy partners doing most of the pedaling and balancing. With an able and able-bodied mate, some can still beat the less skilled at table tennis. When a swimmer discovered he now lacked the strength to maneuver with a scuba tank on his back, he had the scuba tank switched to his chest. That changed his center of gravity and worked fine. So did he. We have more time now to savor what we took for granted—conversation with an old friend, the taste and texture of a hot fudge sundae, the burst of color in a neighbor's garden.

EYE PROBLEMS: Since double vision only bothers you with both eyes open, use a plastic shield, alternately covering one eye and then the other. Check your vision regularly because diplopia is only a temporary symptom. Eye problems should encourage you to develop your memory.

FALLS: Most of us endure bruised knees and cracked ribs until we learn how to avoid falls. We trip over a dropped foot or fail to lift our foot enough to clear a curb or the next step up. We may turn too quickly and lose balance or our legs simply fold and we drop. Many times we fall getting out of bed because our legs stiffen during sleep. A friend who drags a foot finds scatter rugs his worst enemy. After two fractured ribs, he cleared the rugs from his bedroom.

As in skiing, the trick is to fall relaxed. If you cannot easily recover lost balance, just drop. Trying to brace myself as I fell, I suffered a shattered elbow in one fall and a cracked kneecap in another. One woman alone told me she is terrified of falling because she finds it hard to get up. You can meet that problem by lying where you fell long enough to recover from the initial shock and try to determine if you broke any bones. Your pain may be masked by shock so you should get moving while you can. If you are in the middle of the floor and unable to get up without leaning on something, crawl or roll over to a sturdy chair or overstuffed sofa, anything you can use as a ladder from seat, to arms, to back. Be sure to shield whatever hurts from further damage as you crawl. If nothing better offers, you can even pull yourself up on a door-knob.

If you fell relaxed, you probably were spared a break, but if you suspect your pain is more than strain, your doctor prob-ably will want you x-rayed. Despite the stir it might cause in your neighborhood, do not hesitate to call an ambulance—when pain doubles you over, an ambulance is the most com-fortable way to go.

FATIGUE: Because sending nerve impulses across demye-linated areas requires extra energy, we are hit suddenly, un-expectedly, with overwhelming fatigue. Fortunately, as little as ten minutes of total relaxation can restore us. My friends have learned these techniques to meet the fatigue that drains them: One young mother lies down on the floor with her two young ones and lets them crawl over her until her strength returns. A secretary, proud she can still work a full day, drops her clothes anywhere when she comes home and falls into bed. Housewives decide what must be done today, what will keep until tomorrow or next week. If we fail to get home before fatigue hits, we can sit on a bench, a curb, even the floor. This is no time to be choosy.

Some victims arrange with the office nurse to let them take a midday nap. Others adjust working hours to take advantage of their best time of day. To recognize fatigue's insidious approach, try keeping a log for a week or two to record what you do, how long you spend doing it, and how you feel afterward. From that, you can determine what you can take and what costs too much energy. You want to know how much is too much and when to take your ten-minute work break. Look for energy-saving shortcuts and pace yourself, even if it takes days to accomplish what used to take hours. When you have taken care of today's priorities, take care of yourself.

GROOMING: Don't let yourself go, along with your legs. Knowing the importance of that, a husband rigged a gadget to help his bed-bound wife wash and set her hair. A blind girl makes up sightless eyes to look beautiful for her husband. Even when you cannot manage clips to set your hair, you can use large rollers that stay in place without pins or clips because flexible nylon hooks catch and hold the hair around the rollers, which can be used one-handed. Usually, those with the disease look younger than able-bodied friends, probably because they rest more and drink less.

HOUSEHOLD TASKS: Some of my friends have no outside help yet manage to run their households from wheelchair or walker. They have pride in their home and ingenuity. Sometimes husbands and children lend a hand, but women living alone can manage their households without help. Their tricks for coping with a home: Barbara McGrath vacuums from her wheelchair. Where her wheelchair will not go, she leans against a bureau to push the vacuum and, if necessary, crawls with the vacuum. When she wants to sew, her son threads the needle and she puts the foot pedal on the table beside the machine to operate it with her hand. When she needs both hands to hold the fabric while she stitches it, she pushes the foot pedal with her elbow.

To avoid darkness, which makes her wobble and lose her way, Dorothy Jenkins has taped a flashlight on the bar of her walker at knee level. Since she has nobody to put out lights behind her, she switches on her flashlight as she makes sure the door is locked and all the lights are off before she goes to bed.

The laundry presents another challenge for women with multiple sclerosis. Penny Renzi puts all her family's dirty clothes in a pillow case and throws it down the basement stairs, following it with her hands free to hold the rail. Since she has trouble climbing stairs with her hands full, she has to make several trips to keep one hand free for the railing, but she welcomes the exercise. With a cart borrowed from the supermarket, Dorothy Jenkins rolls her wash into her laundry room beside the carport and reads a book until everything is washed and dried. Barbara McGrath carries the clothes in her wheelchair—her perpetual carry-all—and folds the clean laundry on the dining room table. Their methods may vary, but they can produce drawers full of clean, ironed, folded shirts and sheets, linens and lingerie with no help from anyone.

Since women with multiple sclerosis always have to consider step-savers and ways to avoid hauling things up and down stairs, Penny keeps two of everything for housecleaning in her two-level house. That means two vacuums, two brooms, two mops.

Household chores involve men, too, and if they have multiple sclerosis, they also have to make adjustments. A friend of mine uses nails instead of screws because, with his partially paralyzed wrist, he can no longer turn a screwdriver. Another has taught his wife and children how to use everything in the house. Now all of them know how to work the furnace and unplug a drain. People with multiple sclerosis have to plan, use their imagination, and take nothing for granted.

INSURANCE: Victims of the disease want to increase insurance protection for their families, but they know they will never again be able to pass a physical. What to do? One friend now has covered his family and insured his mortgage without taking a physical at all. A letter from his bank offered disability insurance covering his mortgage at a low monthly rate. It was open season—no physical—and he grabbed it. Every time he had an opportunity to buy a life insurance policy without the need of a physical, he signed. He found that if you buy $10,000 and $20,000 policies presented as special introductory offers, you not only escape a physical but also need give only your name, address, and whether you have worked the last sixty days. If you want more protection, you must take a physical and answer all the questions on the insurance form, including the state of your health. By sticking to small policies, he escaped physicals and embarrassing questions and accumulated a large portfolio of protection for his family.

LIMITATIONS: Once I wrote down everything I did from the time I got up until I went to bed for the night. The list of accomplishments was reassuring. On another day, though, I cannot do that much, and if I have any sense—which I do not always have—I should not try. The trick is to stop one step short of hurting yourself or making a bad mistake.

Through trial and error, you discover how much you can do now. You, in effect, diagnose your own capabilities and frankly admit your limitations. Never let anybody do for you what you can do for yourself with a little effort, but never be ashamed to ask for help when you need it.

Several of my friends regularly preside over what can best be described as salons. By monitoring the world via television, talking books, radio, and newspapers with all the time they need to keep up, they become the best-informed people they know. They sparkle with the joy of knowledge. As they pour out tea and conversation, they also take time to listen because they know the best conversationalist is often the best listener. One man in good health visits a woman in a wheelchair two afternoons a week. When someone commented that he certainly was doing a fine thing spending time with a housebound friend, he replied: "You don't understand. She has given me so much. She is a continuing inspiration for me and my family." Others who spend their days in wheelchairs stay by their telephones collecting information for themselves and friends. The sightless woman who committed two hundred telephone numbers to memory knows just where to call if a friend needs legal counsel, part-time maid, a cure for corns. For friends who work, she is the perfect ombudsman, shouldering their problems because she has the time and interest to do it. Women like her learn to stop yearning for an impossible future. They treasure their memories but refuse to let the past pull them down. They live entirely in the present.

This seems to be the recipe that works: Yes, know your limitations but stretch your strength and will to the maximum.

LIVING ARRANGEMENTS: Where they live and how they live can make the difference between barren dependence on others and a life of continued striving and hope. Lives shaken by death or divorce can be patched without total dependence on others. The solution is rarely the same for people like us, but the point is that there are workable solutions.

A mother in a wheelchair was living with a daughter who wanted to leave town. A younger woman in the same apartment complex with a milder case of multiple sclerosis wanted to get away from a roommate given to loud and late parties. Introduced by a mutual friend, the two women promptly joined forces. Since their disabilities vary, they divide household chores to suit. In calling for any service, they have the added impact of two rather than one. The Red Cross shops for two; a case worker visits because there are two to serve; their pooled disability pensions go further.

Both men and women alone are determined to avoid going to live with relatives when disease strikes. One friend has lost the use of everything but an arm. With help from the Veterans Administration, he bought a small house and pays a couple to minister to his needs. He refuses to give up his independence.

A man whose wife divorced him could have gone home to his parents but feared their stifling concern. Besides, he liked his own home. Two university students now live with him rent-free in exchange for leaf raking in fall, snow shoveling in winter, and other heavy work. He enjoys doing the cooking himself.

Several girls I know have their own apartments despite pleas from relatives to come live with them. One argued that attacks come so slowly that she has plenty of time to call for help. Another, who uses a wheelchair, feels secure because her sister calls first thing in the morning and every night to make sure all is well. A man who has lived with the disease through nearly forty years and two marriages now rents a room from a couple who give him the privacy he wants but are nearby and helpful should he fall or need other attention.

Even a nursing home does not have to be the end of the

world. Young people needing constant care may get better treatment there than they would at home because they rapidly become the pets of a staff used to seeing only the aged and infirm. One woman dreaded the prospect of entering a nursing home because, for years, a friend had done everything for her —paid the bills, kept the place clean, cooked, and never left her side except while at work. The woman dominated her world from a bed she never left. When the friend needed an operation, the woman with multiple sclerosis had to enter a nursing home because no one was left to care for her. She would be reluctant to admit it, but it turned out to be the best move she could have made. She spends most of her waking hours now in a wheelchair instead of a bed. She is assigned to answering calls to the home's recreation department. With no telephone in her room, she can make all the calls she likes from the recreation area as long as she mans incoming calls. She takes her new responsibilities so seriously that she never stays long on the telephone herself now. The nursing home has gotten her not only out of bed but out of doors. A recreation aide took her to the local Multiple Sclerosis Society's Valentine party and people she had known only as voices on the telephone came up to greet her. Physically, she is getting better care, too. Instead of being tended by a daily cleanup woman and an occasional visiting nurse, she receives physical therapy and a whirlpool bath every day.

PROGRESSION: A fear that never completely leaves people with multiple sclerosis and their families is the prospect of paralysis, although it does not occur in the majority of cases. One husband learned to live with his wife's progressing disease: "A friend of mine whose wife also has MS told me coping with it wasn't so difficult, that when you swim the river with a boulder on your back, nothing seems difficult," he said. "At first, I thought my friend was feeling sorry for himself. Now I realize what he meant. Each time my wife's disorder progresses, it's so gradual, we adjust a little more. You realize you're able to handle it because you did last time."

PLANNING: Admittedly, planning gets more complicated when you have no idea whether this will be a good day or a lost one, how your body will react tomorrow, and whether it is safe to plan a trip next month. So how can you plan? Every achieving person with multiple sclerosis I know answered the same way: Don't postpone your life.

"Does your method of planning take into consideration how you're going to feel tomorrow?" I asked John Kramer. "No," he replied, "my method is to decide what I want to do tomorrow and go do it."

Gerry Shur, my Justice Department friend, speaks of the future this way: "We don't wait. We make long-range plans but anything that can be done now, we do now. MS has caused us not to procrastinate."

One couple say they would like to travel but they cannot make plans until they know what is going to happen. That is defeatist. My achieving friends say go ahead as if nothing has happened. If they must go into a wheelchair later—which is true in less than half the cases—at least they would have done their traveling now. Even a wheelchair should not change their plans.

Your planning should start with today, this day. Establish your priorities. Plan what you should do and would like to do and get as far down the list as you can. If the weather is humid and threatens rain, you might figure on a rougher day than when the day is sunny and dry. Any day that your legs feel steadier than usual, and your hands have a firmer grasp, plan on doing your shopping, getting back to the sweater you hope to finish by Christmas, making a date for lunch with friends.

Your daily plan must include activity, rest, and exercise. In bed, the activity may be more mental than physical and the exercise more limited, but whatever still moves, you should move. As for the rest when you work, you may not be able to lie down at the office, but you can put your head on your folded arms for a few minutes at your desk or put up your feet on a chair and close your eyes. Plan that as a daily routine and you get more done.

Almost everything we do takes longer. We have to forget dressing in five minutes, gulping breakfast, and running to the corner to catch a bus. Our bodies refuse to work that fast now. So give yourself enough time. Dr. Shanahan Cohen, the New Jersey psychiatrist, gives herself an hour and a half to get going. Since she feels less than steady first thing in the morning, she showers after breakfast. She knows she can no longer run from a sound sleep to the emergency room as she did when she was an intern. Now she takes her time and lasts longer.

READING: Talking books from the Library of Congress are available not only for the sightless but for those who lack strength to hold a book, and your Multiple Sclerosis Society can help you get the service. Prism glasses for the severely immobilized may greatly enlarge their visual world, showing half a page instead of two or three lines. A rubber-tipped pencil or stick held in either the hand or the mouth may aid in turning pages. Dramatizations of great historic periods and productions of great plays are now frequently performed on public television, so you are not reduced to soap operas even when reading becomes difficult.

SHOPPING: Even with wheelchairs and walkers you can manage to market, although it takes planning. Penny Renzi knows she can no longer run to the store every day because her vision bars driving. To get exactly what she needs on her once-a-week market forays, she makes out daily menus and follows them closely. Instead of browsing through stores to buy clothes, she now does much of her clothes buying by mail.

The growth of mail-order shopping has been a particular boon to the estimated one out of ten Americans—some thirty-five million of them—now temporarily or permanently disabled. We can shop by mail for almost all we need but our daily bread and milk. Those self-help gadgets I have cited all come from a mail-order catalogue.* For a forty-cent service charge, we can get all our stamps by mail, too. I am on "preferred customer" terms (meaning, I suppose, that I pay my bills) with half a dozen mail-order houses and a dozen others woo me regularly with catalogues. Most of my coats, cosmetics, dresses, blouses, books, lingerie, and household gadgets come by mail.

Except for food, a bedridden woman with three school-age children does the family shopping by mail. Her husband fills her food order but for all other family needs she uses her well-thumbed Sears catalogue. Although she never leaves bed, she feels an accomplishing part of the family.

On impulse, one woman in a wheelchair tried a gambit that might work for another frustrated shopper. When she tried and failed to get someone to drive her to a curtain sale, she called the store to have the curtains sent out on her charge account. No, she was told, this was a first-come, first-served sale. She would have to come to the store. "But I'm handicapped," she protested. "I have no way to get to your store. I'm living on Social Security, so your sale is important for my budget." The clerk told her it was store policy and hung up. The woman repeated her plea to the store manager. His refusal was even more abrupt. Then the woman, not in anger

---

* Fred Sammons, Inc.; *BeOK* self-help aids; Professional and Institutional Catalogue for 1978; Toll-free Order Phone—800/323-7305; Illinois calls—312/971-0610; or Order by Mail—Box 32, Brookfield, Illinois 60513.

or argument, mused aloud: "I wonder what the President's Committee on the Handicapped would say about your store policy." For a moment, there was dead silence on the line, then: "Give me your name and charge number and I'll see what I can do. No promises, mind." Five days later, the curtains arrived, sale priced.

SMOKING: A longtime smoker gave up cigarettes because they made her unsteadier than she already was. "Smoking went right to my legs," she said. "After a cigarette, I found I had to wait fifteen minutes before I could do any walking." That was not imagination. A highly regarded neurologist says cigarette smoking will temporarily worsen such multiple sclerosis symptoms as stuttering, tremors, stiffness, dimmed vision, and weak muscles.

Aware that cigarette smoking does them more damage than it does to healthy people who have to worry only about their hearts and lungs, smokers with multiple sclerosis take two approaches. One man says, "I have had to give up so much. I'm not going to give up one of the few things I can still enjoy." The other says, "I have fewer ways now to accomplish things. If I can stop smoking after all these years, I will really have accomplished something." And he did.

TELEPHONE CALLS: The telephone is both lifeline and challenge. How can I dial or even use a touch telephone when I cannot see? How can I converse or even know the telephone is ringing when I cannot hear? How can I use a telephone when I cannot hold it in my hand or dial a number? Telephone services are now being developed to answer those questions and many more. A telephone company brochure, entitled *Services for Special Needs,* available from local Bell Telephone business offices, spells out what is now available, and more aids are being devised all the time. At a national multiple sclerosis conference in Washington, a victim dialed a call with a "breath switch," a new device using breath control rather than fingers on buttons or dials. Her hands were in her lap and the telephone was held on her shoulder by a clamp attached to her wheelchair as she breathed into a pipe she held between her pursed lips. She made the call to Senator Edward Kennedy, chairman of the health subcommittee, at his Capitol office. Another version of the breath switch involves a plastic card that the caller blows on to attract the attention of an operator and blows on again to signal the end of the call.

Those who have trouble dialing because of partial paralysis or impaired coordination use a device that stores and dials from sixteen to thirty-two numbers at the touch of a button. When the right button is pushed, the desired number is dialed automatically. Whatever the problem, the local telephone company may have the device or combination of devices to bring you back into the mainstream.

TRAVEL: From being the overlooked, ignored, housebound, the disabled have become the most favored on the travel scene. Hotels that fail to provide sufficient access are losing convention business. We board airplanes ahead of everyone else. We ride airport elevators while the able-bodied wrestle their carry-on luggage up and down stairs.

In many places, when we go to theater, we pay half price for the best seats—on the aisle or in a box. On a bus, we are entitled to front-row seats and any able-bodied persons in our seats must get up when we appear.

Special attention takes many forms. The time my leg was freshly out of a cast when I flew to Florida, I rode a wheelchair from airport to airplane and was met with a wheelchair in Miami. The attendant would have pushed me all the way to the waiting car if I had not asked him to let me out just before I rounded the bend where mother was waiting for me. John Kramer, who would brush off a flight to Teheran as routine before multiple sclerosis ended his transatlantic business, now speaks with genuine enthusiasm about a train ride from Washington to New York. "They really take care of you on the Metroliner," he said. "A man met me outside the station, got me to my train seat and arranged to have me met on arrival. At Penn Station, another man got my luggage out, wheeled me through the station, put me in a cab, and away I went." He and I had both done the one thing that makes superservice possible. We both made advance arrangements.

On Amtrak, the call a handicapped traveler makes to the railroad's toll-free information and reservations number is the key to a successful trip. A reservations clerk can tell you what problems you may encounter in stations and on trains, what special services are offered and what to do to get special arrangements to make your trip more comfortable. Whether you are riding short or long distances, reserved or unreserved, you should call Amtrak a reasonable time ahead of your trip so special arrangements can be made for you. Special seats, a special car, and especially designed sleeping accommodations are all planned to serve the handicapped, and more than sixty train stations have been built or renovated to remove all barriers from handicapped travelers.

If you travel by air, two steps will ensure you the royal treatment. Again, make your reservations well in advance, identifying yourself as a person needing assistance. That ensures that notice of your needs reaches the right people. The other step is an early check-in, giving the airline time to get you aboard and seated comfortably before other passengers.

Traveling by car, you will find these facilities at the more than eight hundred barrier-free rest areas: ramps instead of steps; wide doorways and easy-opening doors; wide aisles and corridors; toilet stalls that can accommodate wheelchairs and have doors swinging out; support bars in the stalls; lowered towel racks and mirrors; water fountains within reach of a

person in a wheelchair; telephones mounted at the proper
height in a barrier-free booth; paved wide sidewalks and
ramped curbs in parking lots and extra wide parking places
reserved for people in wheelchairs. A compilation called
"Highway Rest Areas for Handicapped Travelers" is available
from the President's Committee on Employment of the Handicapped, Washington, D.C. 20210. From the same source,
you can get "A List of Guidebooks for Handicapped Travelers." You can write then to the addresses listed in the cities
you want to visit in the United States, in Europe, Canada and
Australia to get their guidebooks for handicapped visitors.

WALKING: Legs weakened by an attack or slowed by a
dropped foot have to be retaught. The secret of learning to
walk again is simple: Visualize what you are going to do before you do it. Visualizing is a working principle of yoga, but
I heard the same theory expounded by a veteran of forty years
of multiple sclerosis, a graduate of a nursing home, now able
to get around on two canes. How does he do it? "I had to
relearn to walk. I visualize every step before I take it. Nothing happens until I give specific instructions to each foot to
move. Then it moves."

One woman's doctor told her if she took very short steps
instead of her usual stride, she could manage without falling.
What a physiotherapist once advised works better for me:
Keep your hands free as a starter. If you have to carry cash
and passes, stick them in your pocket. Then march, lifting up
your feet and swinging your arms—not way out like a soldier
but only a little way out to give you balance and a feeling of
freedom. With arms a little bent as they swing, left foot, right
arm, right foot, left arm, you have total balance. It helps to
whistle encouragement. The "Colonel Bogey March" from
The Bridge on the River Kwai does nicely. People passing by
may whistle, too.

WEIGHT CONTROL: In multiple sclerosis, where muscles are weakened and activity may be limited, extra pounds add a burden you may not be prepared to bear. Overweight not only wastes precious energy but taxes your muscles further. It also taxes your family if you must be lifted from bed to wheelchair or helped up from a fall. You do not want those closest to you to strain their backs or develop hernias just because they care for you. To be blunt about it, if you ever need to go into a nursing home, you ruin your chances of getting into a good one if you weigh too much. Given a choice between two patients, a nursing home will take the thinner one because that puts less burden on the staff. Excess weight taxes the strength of whoever has to do the carrying, whether nurse or member of the family.

Find out from your doctor what you should weigh, and if it is considerably less than you weigh now, get on a diet and stick to it. The more you exercise, the easier it will be to shape up.

WHEELCHAIRS AND AMIGOS: Deciding to go into a wheelchair is probably the most important decision a person with multiple sclerosis has to make if his disease progresses. Usually he fights it, but once the decision is made, a frequent reaction is relief. No more dragging reluctant legs, no more stumbling around with a cane, no more slow and boring progress with a walker. John R. Brown, my New Zealand friend, considered the battery-operated wheelchair he bought in London on his 30,000-mile world trip as giving him a new beginning. "If I'm not tired," he said, "I walk. When I tire, I get in my wheelchair and I can keep on going." That is one trick of wheelchair life, not to get too dependent on it. If possible, doctors suggest, keep the wheelchair out of the house—in the garage or van where it is available for getting around town but not a continuing temptation to give up all use of the legs.

Anyone who spends all her time in a wheelchair runs the risk of pressure sores called decubitus ulcers unless she changes position often. If possible, a person should get out of the chair to stand for five minutes out of every hour. If you cannot stand, at least change position every fifteen to twenty minutes either by pushing against the chair arms to lift yourself off the seat or by shifting weight from side to side. A seat pad may be helpful and a pad behind your back will force you to sit straighter so you can take fuller breaths.

The wheelchair is not the sole answer for anyone whose legs refuse to do the whole job. The Amigo is now the popular alternative. The sleek, compact, battery-operated three-wheeler, with feet resting on a platform below the seat, was designed specifically for victims of multiple sclerosis—one victim in particular. In 1967, Allan Thieme, a Bridgeport, Michigan, plumbing and heating contractor, decided to give his wife, Marie, "motorized legs" to make up for the ravages of multiple sclerosis. Thieme figured out the specifications, hired an engineer to carry them out, and named the scooter Amigo because the idea came to him on a vacation in Mexico. In some ways, it is better than a car because the six Thieme children never ask to borrow it. "They know it's mom's legs," Mrs. Thieme said.

Since the Amigo requires the ability to sit up unaided, it is not for everybody, says John Kramer, the former supersalesman who says his Amigo brought him back to life. On a trip, he explained, he had reached the point when he could no longer explore with his family because his legs were too weak to carry him through a sight-seeing expedition. At home, he saw his independence evaporating when he constantly had to ask someone else to get him something from the kitchen, answer the telephone, see who was at the door. Now he flips around in his Amigo, indoors and out. The machine is lighter in weight and eight inches narrower than a conventional wheelchair. As 1977 ended, the Amigo won the blessing of Congress when the final version of the Social Security measure was amended to provide Medicare reimbursement for the Amigo. That means added freedom for an untold number of Americans.

WRITING: Your handwriting is going to change as your grip becomes less firm or your hand less steady. Unless your bank knows your problem, you will get calls—as I have—wanting to know if that is really your signature or a clumsy forgery. If you fear your bank will not honor your signature, sign a new signature card and change it every time your writing changes substantially. Or get your signature put on a rubber stamp. If you cannot use your hands, you can hit the stamper with your elbow, jaw, or foot. Do not let someone else sign your checks for you. Be independent. Say, "This is my check, my money, and I will take care of it one way or another."

If you cannot grasp the average pen, you can get one of those inch-thick, multicolored pens that are easier to hold. A midwestern producer of self-help aids, many of which are suggested in hospitals and rehabilitation centers, has several gadgets to hold a pencil between the fingers when the hand no longer performs.

YOURSELF: How well you cope with a world bounded by multiple sclerosis, how far you venture beyond that world, depends largely on yourself. These rules for living, time-tested by my friends, should help:

You must learn to like yourself before anyone will like you.

Don't get mad at yourself when you drop things or wet your pants. It is not your fault, so give yourself a break. Listen to your own body for the best gauge of medicine that helps rather than harms. If you follow a course of treatment that seems to be good for you, it probably is. Laughter is better for you than tears, but cry if you feel like it.

Be independent. The more you do for yourself, the more you can do. Visiting friends you think you can help will take your mind off yourself. Anything you stop doing, you may never do again, so keep on exercising, talking, writing, thinking, loving. Find alternatives for what used to be. If you cannot walk, you can sit and read; if reading is difficult, you can listen. There is always something left.

Keep up with new developments in research. New drugs or surgical procedures may help you. Know the available resources—the Multiple Sclerosis Society both locally and nationally, the President's Committee on Employment of the Handicapped, the White House Conference on Handicapped Individuals, your Department of Vocational Rehabilitation, the Social Security Administration, the Veterans Administration, and the social service agencies in your community.

Unless you enjoy being handicapped, do not use multiple sclerosis as a cop-out from life. Turn outward for the help you need, but turn inward to find ways you can still help yourself.

Chapter 7

Strengthening the Mind and Body

The first time I saw Norma Grimes, she was tottering into Savitri's yoga studio. Indian-born Savitri Ahuja draws most of her students from the ranks of diplomatic, social, and official Washington, but now she had accepted the challenge of teaching multiple sclerosis victims like Norma how to make forgotten muscles work again. This was Norma's first day, and her mother and young daughter eased her to an exercise mat where she lay until class began. Then she struggled to sit up, bracing herself to keep from falling back. Four months later, as a television camera followed her progress, Norma walked across the studio.

That triumphant walk was one lurching step after another; Savitri stayed in front of Norma both to encourage and catch her if she fell. But she completed the walk unaided and she did not fall. Her victory bolstered the confidence of the class. If Norma, the worst case of multiple sclerosis there, could get across the room on her own, certainly they could do more. It was a lesson Savitri hastened to underline, repeatedly reminding the class that Norma practiced at home an hour a day, refused to give up, refused to say "can't" or "couldn't." After that, everyone in the class who used the forbidden words would hurry to apologize and proceed to do what they had just said they could never do.

Dr. James Q. Simmons, recently retired director of medical programs for the National Multiple Sclerosis Society, endorsed her method. "She pushes people, which is probably what they need. Each person should find out what he can do and do it. Usually, those with multiple sclerosis can do more than they think they can do."

Dr. Simmons observed Savitri's class because it was the first in the country solely for victims of multiple sclerosis. Arranged by the National Capital Chapter of the national society, it was intended only as a two-month experiment. The MS yoga class now has completed its second year and was so well attended that on a March day of snow and slippery streets, nine students appeared for class and some had driven up to two hours to get there.

The willingness of the National Capital Chapter to put some of its limited funds into yoga reflects a growing emphasis on exercise. A neurologist will say—as one said to me—that exercise cannot alter the course of the disease. My own doctor— an internist—told me of three cases, however, where his patients, on an exercise regime, were mobile until someone suggested they seek other medical opinions. By the time they returned to him three to six months later each had lost the use of his legs. My doctor does not contend that exercise prevents demyelination of nerve fibers, but he does argue—as he argued successfully with me—that a regular routine can prevent muscles from atrophying, legs from weakening, and both arms and legs from contracting. Some leading authorities on MS believe it may be possible that regular exercise delays deterioration of muscle and nervous systems.

Increasingly, neurologists—and patients, too—are making the point that since the disease affects the nerve fibers rather than the muscles, if we can keep our muscles from atrophying, we will be ready for the cure when it comes. At least, we can forestall any loss of muscle power arising solely from disuse. The exercise routine can apply to people in a wheelchair and even in bed. In fact, I have seen some patients move from wheelchair to walker because of faithful adherence to an exercise regime. Some probably did not belong in wheelchairs to begin with, and exercise showed them there was still life in their legs. Even yoga exercises performed as regularly as Norma Grimes did them cannot make every victim get up and walk again, of course, but any regime approved by a patient's physician to meet that patient's needs will improve breathing, circulation, and—possibly most important of all—independence.

The National Multiple Sclerosis Society stresses the goal of independence in a 1978 manual entitled *Home Exercises* for patients who can walk or walk with aids. Detailed drawings show how to move each part of the body, from head and neck to ankles and toes, in order to maintain and increase muscle strength, particularly in unaffected muscles. Patients are told that by using these physician-prescribed exercises and aids in walking, they will not only be helping themselves to maintain physical fitness but will also be a step closer to achieving a more independent life.

The drive to restore a patient's independence and set him firmly on the road to hope begins—or should begin—in the hospital after the first attack. The physiotherapist becomes the bridge between the active life that was and as active a life as the patient's own determination can make of the future. The physiotherapist at the hospital, and later at home or at the clinic, can help patients recover some range of motion in affected arms or legs, can demonstrate how to use a board to slide from wheelchair to bed or bath, how to start a home exercise program.

The physiotherapist who showed me leg-strengthening exercises and how to walk like a soldier without shuffling my feet also visited Rita Dalton regularly. As both he and Bill Dalton acknowledged, what he could do for her was limited by her helplessness, but he gave her a feeling of life and hope and belonging.

While the physiotherapist gives passive exercises to those whose muscles need outside help, he also readies patients for home exercise and for exercise offered by a local chapter of the society, by the local "Y," by a health club or a swimming club.

Patients less affected by the disease can go into the "Y" programs or health clubs as long as their physician approves their exercise routine and as long as they stay with it. My friend Lois Ryan, after checking with her neurologist, joined a health club led by a degree-holding "exercise physiologist," who directs Lois in exercises designed to strengthen weak muscles while protecting her against the headaches she used to suffer. Lois cautioned against health clubs with expensive long-term contracts but no personnel trained to gear exercises to specific health problems.

Several state chapters of the society offer regular swimming programs with access to pools with electric lifts to get patients safely in and out of the pool, or ramps where patients can wheel their chairs to the water and tumble off to swim. In other places, a cadre of volunteers helps patients up and down easy steps. One Virginia girl told me: "Each week for one hour, my MS disappears as I walk straight, run as hard as I wish, and do my exercises with ease. Freedom comes with a splash when I enter the pool."

The Utah State Chapter launched a swimming program in 1974, not to teach swimming strokes but to build endurance and exercise muscles directly affected by the disease as well as those atrophied through disuse. Since one-third of the body weight is taken away because of the buoyancy of the water, a 180-pound person in chest-high water can function like a 130-pound person. That makes all the exercises easier and accomplishments greater.

At first in Salt Lake City, members of the family joined patients in the pool. That turned out to be a mistake because the swimming period became "more recreational than therapeutic"—they frolicked instead of getting down to the serious business of making unused muscles work again. Since then, family members have watched from poolside as the patients go through a routine of kicking forward, backward, and to the side; swinging their arms; standing on toes and then heels; stretching their shoulders by holding on to the diving board from underneath; doing the back stroke, the flutter kick, or other leg kicks. One patient confided that for the first time in twenty years he was now able to jump and get off his feet.

Because the former golf champion Jeane Hofheimer leaves Washington every winter for an Arizona resort, the hotel there has installed a lift that makes swimming possible for Jeane, whose legs are crippled by multiple sclerosis, and for other visitors who have trouble getting into the water.

Elaine Dewar's husband fitted her out with a mask, snorkle, and fins when—like so many other victims—she could no longer stay horizontal in the water. The fins kept her legs from dropping and the snorkle and mask helped her regain breath control. She learned to swim normally again.

Even without fins and periscope, a person whose legs refuse to work can stay afloat in a bathing suit with an inflatable bust and buttocks, or "floatees," like those wrapped around each arm to support patients in the Utah swimming program, or a waist swimming belt of pieces of Styrofoam that children use to learn to swim. Gradually, as you get closer to your goal of swimming the length of the pool once, then several times, you can discard pieces of Styrofoam until your muscles are performing again.

So great are the advantages of a regular exercise program in the water that Dr. W. W. Tourtellotte, chief of the Neurology Service at VA Wadsworth Hospital in Los Angeles, has prepared with others a comprehensive booklet entitled *Exercise for Life: Hydrotherapy and the Multiple Sclerosis Patient*. In it, he presents a special hydrotherapy exercise program, reviews commercially available home pools and other hydrotherapy equipment, lists the MS literature and even appends an exercise log book.

Water exercises may help more than land exercises for MS patients, Dr. Tourtellotte contends, because benefits can be altered depending on how the exercise is done. For instance, one water exercise of stretching movements can increase flexibility and improve posture while a similar one of "water resistance" movements can build muscle tone and coordination.

Another benefit is that the pool removes excess heat from the patient's body so he can enjoy exercise without the overheating that can decrease muscle function, fatigue him, make him dizzy or even temporarily blinded. Where the patient has his or her own pool, temperature can be controlled to make it right for the patient. For hydrotherapy exercises at home, a pool at least five feet wide and four to six feet deep is required to allow enough freedom of movement to do the exercises (with a life jacket, of course).

Ocean bathing can be great for those with multiple sclerosis because of the buoyancy of salt water if one can cope with the hazards of walking through sand or meeting the waves and undertow. One West Coast resort put a concrete ramp to the water's edge for people in wheelchairs. Without a ramp, a person with multiple sclerosis who usually walks without a cane may need a cane or a friendly arm to plow through. The second hazard, getting knocked down by a wave, has happened to me more than once since my footing, at best, is never too secure, but on one occasion I lost all sense of direction. I was lucky a swimmer was nearby to haul me out. A third hazard is the undertow. Even if you manage to ride a wave into shore, in those last few feet when you try to scramble to your feet the undertow can pull you back and down. The moral: In the ocean, swim with a buddy.

You can adapt your daily life into a continuing exercise regime. The more you go up and down stairs, for example, the stronger leg muscles will get. The more walking is done with arms swinging naturally, legs lifting, knees slightly bent, and shoulders back, the more confidence will return. By standing erect with chest lifted and shoulders free of their usual slump, you will be able to breathe more deeply. Exercise by chewing gum (except at bed-time); foot-tapping for two minutes without stopping; writing fast and neatly. Knit, type, or play music.

Awareness of one's body—its new weaknesses and remaining strengths—must become as important to a person with multiple sclerosis as brushing one's teeth and paying taxes. Yoga—hatha or exercise yoga—can be the vehicle for achieving that awareness. Yoga came into my life more than a dozen years ago after my doctor had told me I had to do knee bends and some form of bicycling to keep my legs from stiffening. A friend gave me a beginner's yoga book, which I duly studied and tried to follow. I did not understand my own body's needs well enough to gear the exercises to meet them. When I heard that a yoga teacher was conducting a class nearby, I investigated. My limp was very slight then, hardly noticeable even to me, and I thought I was doing as well as any of the novices there when Savitri came over to me and said in a voice only I could hear, "I can help you."

Because of her, I do an hour's yoga a day. I know it makes a difference because when I travel and lack the time or space to exercise, my limp gets progressively more noticeable. And sometimes I stumble and fall.

For anyone with multiple sclerosis, hatha yoga can be more helpful than other forms of exercise because:

• If a person cannot stand on his own, he can still gain many benefits from yoga exercises in a sitting or lying position.
• Yoga is one form of exercise that does not overheat (becoming overheated is something we try to avoid). It also relaxes tension and relieves stress, which we must always combat.
• Since yoga involves no competition (except one's personal competition with himself to make each day more meaningful) it can be done at a person's own pace and time.
• Although many yoga exercises are specifically designed to cure certain ills of the type often encountered by those with multiple sclerosis, its stress on breathing and improved circulation are designed to keep the whole body free of ills.
• Planned as a daily program, yoga can reach more muscles, tone more parts of the body than any other form of exercise. Even Dorothy Cox, a devotee of swimming, found yoga got to more muscles than swimming.

After I took off my blinders a few years ago and began my investigation of multiple sclerosis, I discovered how few of my new friends were exercising. Few of their doctors had attached much importance to exercise, or if they did, my friends were not listening. Gerry Shur was rock scrambling and mountain climbing; Dorothy Cox was swimming regularly, and so was Tim Drury; but few others even mentioned exercise to me.

When I told Diane Afes, patient services director of the National Capital Chapter, that Savitri now was teaching yoga to three patients, she took fire. Would Savitri consider teaching a class devoted exclusively to people with multiple sclerosis? Thus began the chapter's two-month experiment that grew into a continuing program, and attracted the interest of television.

Just as no two patients have the same symptoms, no two react the same way to Savitri's yoga. The yoga has helped their backaches, tremor and dropped foot, their bladder and bowels, insomnia, tension, and sex.

One after another, the girls would report that their doctors were well pleased. Anne Jackson said her doctor found her blood pressure lowered, and Savitri explained that was due to the yoga breathing.

Another young woman confided that after she got the disease, she lost all feeling in her groin and all the joy went out of sex. She cried to her husband, "Have I lost that, too?" Now, she said, she could have orgasms again. The exercise that helped her also aids the spine. Lying on your back with knees up, you arch your back—breathing in as your buttocks go up, breathing out as you lower them, three times in succession. Blood circulating to the pelvic area during the exercise can get rid of the numbness that bothered her.

A variation of the same exercise helps weakened legs and a dropped foot. While you have your back arched and you are breathing normally, straighten one leg up and down, without touching your feet to the ground, and return to the original position. Do the same with the other leg—up, down, do not touch, back to place. Try to do it six times before lowering your back to the floor.

Probably Savitri has had her greatest success in the class in dealing with the prime problem of victims—an unpredictable bladder. One girl who used to get up five or six times now sleeps through the night. Knowing she can now control her bladder, she says she feels free to make engagements, go on shopping expeditions, dine out. Now in her thirties, she knows a confidence she has lacked since she was eighteen. The exercise that has helped her and the others in the class is to stand straight, with legs together, and tighten the buttocks. When you do that, your stomach automatically goes in and the muscles in the front of your thighs become as firm as the tightened buttocks. Anyone who holds that position whenever standing up, whether waiting for a bus or washing the dishes, is putting strength back in weakened muscles and controlling the urinary process. All this and better posture, too.

For those to whom constipation has become a problem, Savitri gives this exercise: Fifteen minutes after drinking the juice of half a lemon and half a spoonful of honey in a glass of warm water, prepare to do a stomach lift. That involves taking a breath and then breathing out slowly until as much air as possible has left your lungs. When so much air has been expended that the area just below your rib cage looks caved in, bend your knees slightly and with hands on your thighs, pull your stomach up and in. Still holding your breath, push your stomach out and in as many times as you can before you have to take a breath. Go ahead and have your breakfast. A trip to the bathroom should follow shortly.

When her students complain of insomnia, Savitri tells them to do the "locust" before going to bed. Lying on their stomachs with their arms and legs stretched out, they take a breath while raising straight arms and legs as high as they will go. When they can hold their breath no longer, they slowly lower arms and legs as they breathe out. They are supposed to do that six times to get the same amount of exercise as they would from a one-mile walk. I invariably start yawning on the third round.

Backaches are a constant problem for anyone with multiple sclerosis because of bad posture. We tend to tilt our bodies forward to avoid falls and get one-sided from leaning on a cane or crutch. To ease that kind of backache, stretch out on the floor with clasped hands turned palms out over your head. Keeping your back as flat on the floor as possible, straighten and stretch your arms and legs as far as they will go. Be sure your toes are up and heels pushing out. That will help your dropped foot, too.

Another exercise Savitri's students like to ease the spine and deal with a dropped foot also begins with a back stretch. Lying on your back, stretch your right arm and left leg as far as they will go on a breath. Do the same with your left arm and right foot. Repeat with both arms and both feet. Now stretch your right arm and right foot simultaneously and, finally, your left arm and left leg. You have three things to remember: Keep those heels pushed out to strengthen a dropped foot. Keep your back flat on the floor. Give yourself a good stretch.

Continually, Savitri emphasizes yoga breathing to ease tension, get rid of a false appetite, stimulate thinking, lower the blood pressure, power the body. She tells her students to breathe out very slowly, as if they were letting the air out of a balloon, and then breathe in to fill the balloon. The breathing is not from the chest but from the diaphragm. "People in wheelchairs," she tells the wheelchair members of her MS class, "cannot increase their circulation by jumping around. I want you to put the emphasis on breathing. Your body needs oxygen to go to every blood vessel."

Now she tells them to close their eyes and visualize the weakest part of their bodies. "Take a deep breath and say that part is getting warmer. Think only of that part. While you are breathing in, you are warming that part. You are giving it life. Oxygen is doing that to you. At first you may not feel it. . . ."

A girl interrupted. "I feel it getting hot."

Savitri nodded. "When you exercise, I want you to use that part. Breathe in and pick up that arm and feel your blood working on that part."

She watched a girl sitting on the mat, struggling in vain to lift her leg even an inch. Finally, she said, "Think what you're doing. Feel that foot. You *like* that foot. Move it. Feel it. Relax. Talk to your foot. Now pick it up." And the girl did.

Repeatedly, she tells her class: "You don't do anything in

yoga without thinking. Think, visualize, feel. Tell yourself, 'I'm going to do this.' " To a woman staring dismally at her lifeless leg, she said, "Don't look at your leg. Feel it. Pick up the easy leg first. That will give you encouragement to pick up the other one."

She is variously tough and tender, encouraging and chiding. When a woman climbed out of her wheelchair and shouted, "I'm standing," Savitri retorted, "Of course, you are. What's the big deal about that? I told you you would stand." What the woman failed to realize was that Savitri wanted more from her. "Now, move. Take a deep breath and get straight like a young girl. Feel young. Now take a step. You see, your foot is moving." The woman took a tentative step and smiled triumphantly before she started to topple. "Next week," Savitri told her as she helped her recover her balance, "I want to see you walk over to that post." The woman stared at the post— it could have been a mile away but she did not say, as she had been saying for weeks, that she couldn't do it.

When the students complain of aching muscles, Savitri tells them: "Be glad you ache. That means you're using muscles you haven't used in a long time. When your muscles come to life, they give you pains and aches which you should love."

When Mildred Smith's minister son brought her to class in a wheelchair and carefully lifted her into a straight chair, Savitri told her, "You don't need a wheelchair, and next week I want to see you on an exercise mat like the rest of them." Mildred Smith believed her. Next week, she appeared with a walker, and this time her son helped her to get down on the floor. In the weeks that followed, Savitri worked on the arm Mildred Smith thought was totally useless. "You have two arms," Savitri told her. "Use them." The right arm went up easily. The left arm moved maybe two inches from her side. "More," said Savitri, "a little more. It's going up."

Mildred Smith looked wonderingly at her bad arm. "Did I

hear you say you couldn't do it?" Savitri asked.

"I surprised myself," the woman admitted sheepishly. The next week when she came to class, she reported a triumph. "I put on my hat myself," she said. "Soon, I'm going to dress myself, even put on my panty hose."

When the class broke up for the summer, Mrs. Smith told me she had gotten more out of her few months of yoga than out of years of private physiotherapy. "I don't put down the physical therapy I have been having. That's what kept me on a certain keel, but if I had been taking this yoga I think I would have grown a little more mentally and physically. I feel yoga is just as necessary as your needles or your vitamins and medication. It becomes a matter of determination. I was determined I wasn't going to use a wheelchair, as she said. I think if I'm determined enough I will get away from it entirely."

She said Savitri was always telling her not to rely only on her strong side but to work the weak side, too. "Last night, my son visited me with his new baby girl. He put the baby in my lap and I tried to hold her and give her a bottle. It fell from my hands but I tried again. I said, I'm not going to give up anymore."

Two of Savitri's students with multiple sclerosis have demonstrated the effect of their yoga in a hospital setting. When Joanne Bell was hospitalized for a pelvic operation, she joined a group of women being briefed the night before on what to expect. The day after the operation, when the women met again, Joanne was the only one able to stand up straight, although she was also the only one with multiple sclerosis. She attributed that to muscles strengthened by yoga exercises.

After Alma Gaghan lost her husband she plunged into his contracting business and, just as I had feared, her overwork and anguish combined to bring on an attack of the disease. In the hospital, with her balance off and her legs feeling

pressure like tight bandages, she spent hours a day at physiotherapy. She learned how to walk again, how to strengthen
her weakened leg muscles by sitting on the edge of a large
ball and moving her pelvis like a belly dancer. When she
stopped rotating her hips, she got down on a mat and did the
bicycling that Savitri had taught her, thrusting a leg straight
out and bringing it back in a bicycle motion but slowly pedaling downward and back up again to strengthen her stomach
muscles. She said the doctors heartily approved the yoga exercises she demonstrated for them.

Savitri is unique in her background of a family of doctors,
her experience as the wife of a diplomat, the varied physical
problems of students she solves, and her own yoga concepts.
Nevertheless, every major American city and many smaller
ones now have at least one yoga teacher with enough training, even self-training, to guide students through a course. If
a person with multiple sclerosis knows his own body's weakness, a yoga teacher with any know-how at all should be able
to tell him which exercises will strengthen.

A class atmosphere helps a multiple sclerosis group because
of mutual support and encouragement. But if no yoga teacher
is available, you can still benefit from yoga exercises by following daily programs on some television stations—particularly public television—or studying a basic yoga exercise book.

Then, as Savitri says, "When you feel every day you are
doing better, that's your life. That's hope."

Chapter 8

Doctors Neither Gods
nor Villains

Elaine Dewar was sleeping away so much of the day that her two-and-a-half-year-old had to mind the baby. The doctor called her overwhelming urge to sleep "housewives' syndrome" or "the seven-year itch." He did not connect it with her earlier episodes of pins and needles shooting down her right leg.

He put her in the hospital finally, but all she got out of that was a prescription for tranquilizers. Thus began Elaine's long search for the truth of her condition. Her eyes were hit next. She noticed that her left pupil looked smaller than her right, and when she tried to catch a ball, she reached for it before it arrived. An eye specialist found nothing wrong, but then a gray shade began to descend over her left eye and she went temporarily blind. A burning sensation on her upper thigh got so intense she had to cut off her pants leg because she could not bear anything touching her skin.

For the first time, she was sent to a neurologist who hospitalized her but afterward told her only, "By the way, you don't have a brain tumor." The eye specialist was now blaming her woes on a high cholesterol count; however, the neurologist, still seeking answers, sent her to a New York hospital for another battery of tests. There, a specialist presented her to his class as a typical case of optic neuritis. When a student asked her if she had a tingling in her arms and legs, the doctor interrupted to say, "No, no, this is a typical case," and hustled the student away while Elaine was saying yes, she did have a tingling. Before she left the hospital, she was told she had a nerve inflammation prednisone would clear up. She was not told that prednisone is often prescribed to reduce nerve inflammation in multiple sclerosis.

Her husband was transferred from Connecticut to Washington, where a neurologist recommended by her family doctor back home also prescribed prednisone. When she asked what was wrong, he replied that the name of the disorder was unimportant. Elaine, who had been a medical technologist before her marriage, studied a family medical guide and told her husband her trouble sounded like multiple sclerosis to her. He promptly called the neurologist to confirm their suspicions and was told, "It's a demyelinating disorder of that nature." Since "demyelinating" was not listed in her layman's book she was stumped again.

The neurologist had recommended that Elaine get a general practitioner. When she told the new man that she was getting up six or seven times during the night to go to the bathroom and had a pulling, curling sensation in her arm, he diagnosed it as a circulatory problem and instructed her to come in three times a week for B-12 shots. In August 1973, while the family was vacationing in Vermont, Elaine found that her right side had stiffened. Enjoy yourself and forget it, the family doctor advised by phone. By now, her right arm felt so frozen, despite a heat wave, that she wrapped a heating pad around it and watched beads of sweat form while she shivered with chill.

Back in Washington, Elaine decided to go to the neurologist who had been originally recommended by others in New York but too busy to see her earlier. He ended her doubt—at least for the moment. He wrote to tell her family doctor that she had multiple sclerosis. After spelling out her symptoms in neurological terms, he concluded: "She is aware of the diagnosis and accepts it with relative equanimity." The family doctor, however, refused to accept it. He put her in the hospital, gave her a spinal tap, and then agreed she did indeed have the disease.

About then, the Dewars moved to a suburban home and to a new doctor who did not believe she had multiple sclerosis. He relied on acupuncture for relief of her symptoms. By the third treatment, Elaine was in such distress that she was sent to a neurologist in a nearby medical building. It was the turning point in her struggle with doctors and disease. The new man confirmed the earlier MS diagnosis and showed her how to bring herself back. He told her to play the piano and type to restore flexibility to her numbed fingers and ignore it when she struck the wrong chords or the type jumbled. He urged her to squeeze a ball to strengthen her forearm, to clap her hands in front and behind her back to regain coordination and to stop her arms from flying around. He told her to practice writing, because she had forgotten how to hold a pen. He would throw coins on the desk and tell her to pick them up. "I used to practice picking up coins at home, hoping that some time I would pick up his quarter and put it in my pocket, but I never got quick enough.

"He was always there when I called him and he didn't rush me off the phone. We'd chat a bit and he always listened, always told me to call when I felt like this. I'd never had a doctor like that before." What probably helped most, though, was his repeated reminder to try to do more on her own. That not only brought back her lost confidence but helped her face the future. Knowledge is the key to Elaine's equanimity.

Physicians often say they tell their patients the facts but the patients do not listen, or, listening, do not understand or exaggerate or forget the facts. Elaine did not forget because years ago, when her husband's work took them to different cities, he started keeping a record of her doctors, hospitals, symptoms, so she would be able to answer a new doctor's questions. Her difficulties, therefore, are documented.

Until recently, almost everyone I met with the disease had a story to tell about doctors, usually negative.

Some had been subjected to unnecessary operations that did not help, or had narrowly escaped operations that could have done harm. They said doctors told them the name of their disorder did not matter when what they wanted most was a name for the unknown. Some complained that when they finally heard the truth, doctors were callous in the telling and brusque, either not taking time to answer questions or frightening them with information they had not requested and did not want. A neurologist told a girl studying for her Ph.D. that she would not go blind or need a wheelchair. Since she had not even considered either possibility, what he may have thought reassuring terrified her. Others said nurses and interns had blurted out the truth before they were prepared to hear it.

Rita Dalton entered the hospital for a month of intravenous injections and was kept in bed the whole time despite the stiffening effect of no exercise. "She walked in," her husband said, "but we brought her out in a wheelchair. She has never walked since then. When you lose it, you don't gain it back." Another woman told me she was put in a wheelchair when she broke her wrist. Her arm healed while her legs stiffened and she has never left the wheelchair. She blames her limitations on "medical action" rather than progress of the disease.

The doctor-patient relationship is beginning to change. But the change is gradual. Some older doctors still refuse to tell their patients the truth, preferring to let a relative make the decision for them. Some younger doctors are too busy to give patients the information and attention they crave when they need it most. Simply telling them to go home and lead as normal a life as possible is hardly enough.

Some doctors realize now that the process of reaching for hope should begin before patients leave the hospital after their first attack. To achieve that, these doctors take a team approach to treatment. Aware that they lack both time and expertise to meet all a patient's newly acquired needs, they bring in a social worker to inform a patient about community resources and a physiotherapist to exercise affected muscles before they wither and to demonstrate how remaining muscles can be strengthened to make the patient as independent as possible. Sometimes, the doctor arranges for an occupational therapist to show a stricken housewife how to continue running her household by reorganizing her tasks and equipment to conserve precious energy. A physician himself may alert the local Multiple Sclerosis Society or tell the patient he or she has somewhere to turn for more information, for advice, and an opportunity to meet others in the same situation. That may not mean much at first, but it will later when former friends slip away and the patient feels a rising desire to see how others have dealt with this turning point in their life. The society may be asked by a member of the hospital team to provide a hospital bed or a wheelchair for the homecoming or to brief the family in advance on what the patient needs. Before the patient leaves the hospital, a caring doctor may also write a prescription for a visiting nurse to come to the home regularly to do for the patient what he cannot do for himself, at least for a while.

A look at even the recent past shows why patients are ready to welcome any change. A thirty-eight-year-old divorcée, working full time to raise four children, for years suffered bouts of numbness, great fatigue, blurred vision, and a staggering gait yet psychiatrists told her the problem was emotional. The physician who finally made the diagnosis in September 1977 figured she had had the disease for ten or fifteen years. An Army wife said her trouble started when her husband was in

Vietnam and her six-month-old baby was hospitalized with a respiratory infection. "The stress probably brought on the attack," she said, "but it took two years before I finally found a doctor who would pay attention to me instead of just handing me tranquilizers."

One man I know had been stumbling and staggering around for six to eight months, wetting his bed, and forgetting his wallet on an airplane, when his doctor-brother arranged for him to see a neurologist. The brother asked the neurologist to tell him the diagnosis. The neurologist honored the commitment to speak to the brother, not the patient. As far as I know, the man still has not been told he has multiple sclerosis. His wife is frantic, but the brother refuses. Probably somehow, someday, she will get the courage to do her own telling.

When doctors hesitate, sometimes the telling is done for them. After a series of incidents, Michael Rubin, of the Justice Department, was hospitalized for tests. One day he watched Frank Sinatra on a television spot announcement to raise money for multiple sclerosis research.

"He seemed to be talking about me, about losing my eyesight and the numbness and not being able to walk. I shouted, 'That's me. I know he's talking about me.' " When the doctor and a nurse tried to brush off his questions, he found his own answer. On the windowsill, he discovered a urinalysis container and the tag on the bottle said, "MS."

Rita Dalton was told by mistake. The doctor had informed her husband but suggested that she not be told until he confirmed the diagnosis by further tests. While the doctor and the husband were talking in the hall, a young intern stopped by Mrs. Dalton's room and told her.

Just as Barbara McGrath discovered what she had by reading her medical chart while riding to therapy, so an Indianapolis girl tilted her head to read the chart hanging on the back of her wheelchair and saw "suspicion of multiple sclerosis."

She thought she was dying. Another woman told me she was actually handed the chart and told to walk it to x-ray. Naturally, she looked to see what it said about her. It said, "This can only be MS." She was discharged from the hospital without being told the diagnosis, so she called the Multiple Sclerosis Society to find out what the disease was all about.

One woman I know discovered just how callous a young doctor can be. She went to Mayo Clinic from her rural Minnesota community when her own doctor would not or could not tell why she was having such trouble walking. "A young resident laid it on the line," she said. "He didn't know me, didn't know I had known nine people with MS in my hometown, including two who died of it. He just said, 'You have multiple sclerosis. I'm sorry there's nothing we can do.' "

Patients in other hospitals speaking of other doctors told similar stories, and the National Advisory Commission on Multiple Sclerosis created by Congress to determine the best way to find the cause, cure, and treatment of the disease obviously had heard those stories, too. In its 1974 report, the commission said that far too often the first professionals dealing with multiple sclerosis patients tell them there is no cure and no treatment of the disease. The commission found these doctors "needlessly negative and harmful."

At least a dozen people told me their doctors, soon after their illness had been diagnosed, advised them to get reconciled to a wheelchair. Every one I met who had heard the wheelchair warning reacted with shock, anger, and a bitter determination to prove the doctor wrong. Later, they may be grateful to get off dragging legs, but telling them at the wrong time, and too soon, can drag them down more than wobbly legs.

Sometimes, though, the anger has been the catalyst for keeping them on their own two feet. Marilyn Pollin said her doctor advised her to get a wheelchair and roll around the house in it until she learned how to use it on the street. "The neurologist told me, 'You're never going to lick it. Stop fighting it.' I'm so glad my husband heard it." Her husband, a psychiatrist and psychoanalyst who directs research for the National Institute of Drug Abuse, said to her, "Let me tell you, the guy is all wet." Marilyn agreed with him. "I have no intention of giving up, I have too many things to do with my life."

Wheelchair arguments are merely symbolic of barely concealed friction between many neurologists and their patients, a friction no doubt heightened by a realization shared by doctor and patient that the disease still eludes a cure. The patient has been brought up to think of a doctor as the infallible healer, just as he appears on television. The doctor, programmed the same way, feels frustrated when the healer's role is denied him. He may become surly and short-tempered when patients repeatedly ask him questions he cannot answer. Some may even order a patient in tears to leave their office. Several patients described such scenes to me.

The cruelest story I heard, though, was told me by Sylvia Lawry of the National Multiple Sclerosis Society. She said that in 1936, when the neurosurgeon to whom she had taken her brother completed his tests and sentenced the boy to an early death, the boy was left in such a state of shock that he urinated all over the doctor's fancy carpet, the first occurrence of the symptom of bladder disturbance. Beside himself with rage, the doctor ordered the brother and sister to get out of his office. "The medical profession's perspective is different now," Sylvia Lawry commented.

The first stumbling block to an effective relationship between doctor and patient is diagnosis. In the past, a doctor has often taken five years or more to decide the patient has the disease, and even then he might have changed his mind. The Mayo Clinic cited two studies showing that doctors took from five and a half to seven and a half years from first symptom to final diagnosis. Doctors still wait to rule out every other disease, especially those that might respond to a specific treatment or those for which there is a cure. If the first sign happens to be an eye problem, as is often the case, the family doctor might simply send the patient to an eye specialist whose tests reveal nothing. Neither the general practitioner nor the specialist may consider multiple sclerosis.

The second sign may appear years later as a dropped foot, and even if a neurologist is called in at that point—which may be unlikely—the episode of the eyes might be long forgotten and not even mentioned. My Aunt Sara Podell recalls that maybe thirty years ago she would tease her husband that he had married a cheap drunk because she could see double without taking a drink. Many years later, after frequent trips to specialists for recurring ailments that left her weaker but no wiser about what was wrong with her, she happened to ask her son to examine her eyes to see if her glasses needed changing. When he finished the examination, he told her gently, "Mother, I think you should have a checkup." Her doctor said it was not necessary, but her son insisted on a spinal tap. Thus, it took an intern fresh from medical school rather than her Park Avenue specialists to diagnose the disease that ultimately put her in a wheelchair. His medical training had been recent enough to make him more alert to the possibility of multiple sclerosis than his mother's contemporaries were. Nowadays, more doctors are aware that eyes telegraph the presence of multiple sclerosis probably more often than any other part of the body. In the absence of any laboratory test that would ensure an accurate diagnosis every time, though, even the best informed, most alert physicians want more than one symptom, however revealing, before they will commit themselves. Usually, that takes more time.

A new international trend favors making a diagnosis within a year. Dr. Helmut H. Bauer of West Germany, whose *Manual on Multiple Sclerosis* was issued in 1977 under the auspices of the International Federation of Multiple Sclerosis Societies and its medical advisory board, is pushing for early diagnosis, even as early as the first bout of the disease. He argues that the cause of multiple sclerosis must ultimately be found in the patient and that the early forms of the disease hold the greatest promise of yielding a clue. He notes especially that doctors should make careful followup observations of all cases of optic neuritis. Aside from the value to research, he believes that doctors might get clues to what the future holds for their patients if the first year of the disease is carefully observed.

Early diagnosis also can launch a patient sooner on the exercise regime that may keep him on his feet and out of a wheelchair.

Dr. Kurtzke believes that patients usually should be told soon. "As a generalization," he said, "the earlier you know what's wrong with you, the better off you are. For one thing, a fair number of people are accused of being lazy or drunk or awkward or negativistic or crocks when it's nothing but MS. So if it's no more than to get these people off the patient's back, I think the patient should be told once a diagnosis is as certain as it can be.

"I have never regarded the diagnosis of multiple sclerosis the way they have regarded the diagnosis of inoperable cancer." In the old days, the doctor would tell the family or tell some other responsible person as he would if the patient had cancer.

Dr. Kurtzke said a doctor will not tell some patients if he thinks they will go to pieces and begin to make a will.

"Isn't it possible," I asked, "that doctors underestimate the mental strength of their patients?"

He said there are depressive reactions and, in rare cases, even suicides among multiple sclerosis victims. I found that while many may reach the brink of suicide, they rarely tip over. In the one suicide I investigated, I strongly suspected that a wandering husband rather than a progressing disease was responsible. A psychiatrist who has been helping patients with multiple sclerosis and their families for ten years agreed with my findings. She said suicide thoughts occur to most of these patients but they are not acted on. In the two cases she knew, they committed suicide because of a philandering spouse.

The implication that she might kill herself probably made Anne Jackson, the brilliant black girl, angrier than anything that had happened since the door at the Washington Technical Institute fell on her head. "The doctor insisted that my family not tell me I had MS," Anne said. "He thought I didn't have the stamina, that I would commit suicide. He didn't realize that I had been raised in a very religious atmosphere, that I would never take my own life."

Dr. Kurtzke explained that the teaching of doctors until the last twenty years advised against telling patients what was wrong. They assumed death would occur within ten years. "It was standard medical school teaching that you didn't tell somebody about a condition you couldn't do anything about." In addition, the diagnosis could be in doubt because other diseases had some similar symptoms. "When you have to come up with a label that you yourself have thought was a death sentence, you don't give it prematurely—not until you're forced to." Dr. Kurtzke said the past medical view of MS was "warped." For older clinicians, he said, it may not have changed. Nowadays, it's more likely the patient will be told, once the doctor is convinced.

The patients I asked were unanimous in wanting to be told, just as they were more than twenty years ago when the National Multiple Sclerosis Society polled its membership about the matter and got an overwhelming Yes vote. Eileen Quick said, "Knowledge has a positive effect. You do things with more fervor." Donna Matzureff, who went ten years without being told, said, "Not knowing is the worst hell of all."

Pauline Schultz, the nurse now in happy remission, opposes any effort to withhold the diagnosis because "by knowing, I was able to alter my life-style and possibly alter the course of the disease." Aware of her disease, she knew she needed a proper diet, exercise, and constant effort to avoid colds and infections. Knowing she must stay out of bed, even after an operation, even after having children by natural childbirth, she was on her feet in a few hours. The doctors said she would never make it, but after her condition was diagnosed, she finished school and had two children.

The truth was kept from the golfer Jeane Hofheimer for many years, and though Jeane is a thoroughly upbeat, non-complaining doer, she feels strongly now that she could have planned things differently if she had known. "If I had been aware of all the things that could trigger an attack," she said, "I would have avoided them. In a golf tournament, if I had known that eighteen holes was enough for me, I wouldn't have gone back after lunch and played another eighteen holes. I would have said no. If I had known that cold air blowing on me wasn't good for me, I wouldn't have slept under an air-conditioning unit and woken up with my whole right side numb, or driving back from Maine I wouldn't have had a cold-air vent pushing a stream of chilly air against one leg and foot for seven hundred miles. I lost all feeling in my right leg and had to be treated with cortisone." It took eight weeks for the leg to function again.

Knowing has prompted some to launch themselves on new careers. Others have begun families. Some girls have decided to have their babies now while they can still take care of them

—just in case they might not be as able to do so later.

Dr. Simmons, former director of medical programs of the National Multiple Sclerosis Society, while acknowledging that patients want to be told, and believing that most should be told, argued nevertheless that doctors should have some options. "Suppose a patient is getting along very well and as soon as she finds out she has the disease and tells her boss, he says, 'We have to find a replacement for Emily.' It all depends on the personality of the individual, whether he or she can take it. As long as the doctor tells somebody in the family, it may not be necessary or wise to tell the patient. Some patients are emotionally unstable for reasons that have nothing to do with MS. Supportive therapy might be advisable before the diagnosis is revealed."

So great are the pitfalls of not knowing that one patient even applied for voluntary admission to a mental hospital because she was sure her mind must be going, until somebody finally told her the truth. What not even doctors may realize is that this unpredictable disease can produce unpredictable reactions. The old idea of doctors handing patients a pill and telling them to rest off their discomfort simply does not work with people who want more than anything else to know the cause of their discomfort. If doctors are going to play the omniscient role, their patients want them to be truly omniscient. Dr. Bauer, the West German authority on multiple sclerosis, said an evasive answer may prompt the patient to conclude that the doctor either does not know what the disease is or that the prognosis is so bad he does not want to reveal the whole truth. He argued that suspense and uncertainty cause far greater stress. The delay, he said, makes the disease that much more ominous and terrifying.

As a marriage and family therapist in addition to patient, Marilyn Pollin feels strongly that patients should be told as soon as the doctor knows. She was outraged after a neurologist patted her on the head and told her to go home and relax, that nothing was wrong. But he told the truth to a psychiatrist she had consulted, who told Marilyn's husband, who told Marilyn that she had multiple sclerosis. She has this view of how patients feel when truth is denied them: "You despair. You think you're irrational. You lose confidence in yourself and in your own mind. When we lose self-confidence, we lose our balance in more than a physical way. Not telling is making a life choice for another human being, and doctors are not gods."

How patients are told, however, may be as important as the telling.

Robert Douglas, who was a virologist at the National Institutes of Health before his illness, believes the doctor should be slow and sure about spreading knowledge of the patient's condition so he and his relatives can absorb it gradually. "It's bad to spring the diagnosis on you and your family immediately," he contended. "People around you aren't sure about the disease. They think it will kill you or make you a vegetable. If you have a long undiagnosed case, in a year you and your family will have gotten conditioned to the fact you have something. By then, you and they want to know."

As psychiatrist as well as patient, Dr. Kathleen Shanahan Cohen wants patients told all that is known about the disease in terms they can understand. She emphasizes that patients should be given plenty of opportunity to ask questions and to call back later with more questions if they have them. "I think they should be told in relatively gentle terms, if it happens to be pretty serious, approximately what their hurt status is and the prognosis also given in gentle terms because, in the first place, we don't know, and also, there are so many variations of the disease.

"The more a doctor can tell you about what is and isn't so about the disease, the better off the patient will be. The doctor should suggest that you will have good days and bad days, but you'll have more good ones than bad ones, so as long as you don't let the bad ones throw you and put you into such a panic that you make yourself worse, you'll be okay. That's what the doctor can do."

From talking with doctors and physiotherapists, staffs of local multiple sclerosis societies, and especially the patients themselves, I found how much doctors can do now to make these once neglected patients the active, contributing people their brains entitle them to be. Everyone I talked with, including the doctors, agrees that the doctor's own attitude toward the disease can make all the difference in both the patient's attitude and motivations. A doctor's outspoken pessimism may drive patients to charlatans with magic cures and to questionable remedies suggested by well-meaning friends. Part of the doctor's negative approach simply comes from lack of current knowledge. One doctor said if his fellow practitioners would only read some medical textbooks published since they went to school, they would lose some of the pessimism that depresses them and their patients. "They only see the severe cases in hospitals," he said. "They don't see the ones riding around on bicycles."

Doctors no longer have to feel frustrated or guilty or helpless. Until they can cure, they can play the role of healer in many ways. More than one patient has told me that, during hospitalization after a bad attack, she found her miserable symptoms beginning to fade after a doctor took the time to sit by her bed and simply talk with her, talk of how she could meet and beat the disease in the way she lived.

A hospital study has established that a placebo, a meaningless medicine, combined with tender loving care, can suffice to make some patients with multiple sclerosis improve. Dr. Simmons noticed similar improvement in a "significant number" of patients who volunteered for research projects even

though all they received was a placebo. The idea that someone cared enough to do research into their disease and that
the project just might be hopeful made them feel better. The
psychological effect proved more effective than any medicine.
More doctors are realizing now that until they find a medicine
that works on the disease itself, all they have to offer—besides
treatment of side effects—is genuine interest in their patients'
well-being!

Instead of leaving him to feel rejected, isolated, and worth-
less, the doctor can give the patient the impression that he
and his family are part of the healing team. Then, instead of
hating—even blaming—the doctor, the patient will know that
if anything can be done, they will do it together. Just showing
that someone cares may be all the reassurance a patient needs,
but the doctor can also leave the door wide open to hope by
stressing the possibility of lasting remissions, a benign course,
and the promise of research. The doctor will make it plain that
he cannot predict what the future will bring but he can refer
to Dr. Kurtzke's study of World War II veterans and its finding
that the severity of a patient's disability five years after onset
of the disease is likely to be the way it is twenty years later. In
Dr. Kurtzke's twenty-year study, two-thirds of the patients
kept the same neurological function they had five years after
the first attack and the other third were only slightly worse.
Soon, Dr. Kurtzke will have completed analyses of how veterans with the disease fared thirty years later, and that should
provide more reassurance—at least more certainty, and uncertainty sometimes is the hardest thing to bear.

The doctor can make sure he has answered questions fully
so his patient will keep away from obsolete and terrifying
health books. Gerry Shur, my Justice Department ally, had
approached his problem as the lawyer he was, researching
and briefing. "You read this stuff and it's absolutely devastat-

ing. You read you're going to be crippled, confined to bed
with neither bladder nor bowel control. You'll never see again,
you'll mumble. Physically, you may get better but from reading that stuff, you remain scared." His "research" led to
despair not to hope.

Robert Douglas, no stranger to the disease from his years
at NIH, advised: "Tell people to close the MS textbooks. They
show a little bit of knowledge can be dangerous." Dr. Uhlmann agreed. He said the neurologist friend who gave him
the diagnosis also told him not to read a lot of articles by
experts who really have no answers. Dr. Bauer said giving a
patient the information he needs (rather than forcing him to
seek it in obsolete tomes) "may be time-consuming, but in
many cases it is the most important help a doctor can give his
patient."

Ann Krasnicki, the CIA employee, wishes her doctor had
taken the time to tell her the disease could be cyclical. If she
had known that, she said, she would never have given up her
apartment and gone home to Pittsburgh when the disease
struck. As it was, she returned to the CIA when she recovered
and had to go through the business of finding another apartment.

The most hopeful advice I found being given by a doctor
to doctors about how patients with multiple sclerosis should
be treated was offered by Dr. Wallace W. Tourtellotte, chief
of the Neurology Service at the Veterans Administration
Wadsworth Hospital Center in Los Angeles, vice-chairman of
the neurology department in UCLA's School of Medicine, and
author of hundreds of medical treatises.

To start doctors thinking about their patients in terms of
hope rather than defeat, Dr. Tourtellotte advises: "If we help
them to live as fully as possible, they will be able to cope with
most aspects of their grim disease. Accordingly, they will be

in the best possible mental, physical, and neurological health to receive the coming of the as yet undiscovered treatment."*

Like Dr. Kurtzke, he believes the patient should be told he has the disease only when it is definite. Since many times a suspicion of the disease is not borne out by later developments, he tells his patients they have "neuritis" and further tests are needed. He will talk to them about a virus infection of the brain and suggest that body defenses are fighting the virus. If neurological signs or symptoms appear, he will say they may be due to scars in certain control centers. But he never mentions multiple sclerosis until he is sure. Then, he said, he tells the patients, but he makes these qualifications: There is no way of proving the diagnosis but the patient's neurological history and signs, possibly the results of a spinal tap, and tests ruling out other disease make it the most probable diagnosis. He will tell them laboratory tests may be repeated at intervals to verify the diagnosis. Since the state of a patient's health cannot be predicted, he recommends an examination every nine months to a year. He tells patients that, in his experience, most patients have mild to moderate disease with long remissions. He illustrates with a few case histories. He reassures them that the fearful impression of the disease they have gotten from seeing a bedridden or wheelchair-bound patient is not the average case. He encourages patients to talk with him about their illness rather than to learn about it from laymen's literature. He stresses that since the disease rarely affects a patient's memory or thought processes and rarely produces pain or depression, a patient can still set goals for himself.

Recognizing their concern about the future, Dr. Tourtellotte tells patients the average life expectancy with this disease is just short of that for others of the same age group. And he

* *Clinical Neuropharmacology*, Vol. 2, edited by H. L. Klawans, chapter 9, "Therapeutics of Multiple Sclerosis." New York, Raven Press, 1977.

finds it reassuring to mention Dr. Kurtzke's five-year rule—
the severity of your condition five years after onset is the way
you are likely to be twenty years later. If the patient asks,
Dr. Tourtellotte says, he should be told periodically that his
condition might worsen and he should report any significant
change so a decision can be made as to whether further tests
or a change in treatment is warranted. Because these patients
are particularly sensitive to the stresses of daily living, Dr.
Tourtellotte says their physicians have to be ready to give
advice on everything from anesthesia for pulling a tooth (no
problem, he says) to megavitamins and special diets (the
money would be better spent, he says, on a donation to
multiple sclerosis research).

While the medical problems of people with multiple sclerosis are being met with increased efficiency, some patients—
including doctor-patients—would like to see more emphasis
on treating the total patient, the total family, his total problem. One of the most vocal is Dr. Panzarella. "They will treat
the patient for his acute illness, but once that's over, they're
either afraid or indifferent to the needs a patient may have in
the psychological, social, and vocational areas." He contended that doctors don't pay heed to the person's needs as a
member of a family, as a member of society, whether he can
return to work and, if not, whether some agency can be
found to help get him back to work. "This requires a tremendous amount of time and effort, and most doctors don't
have that kind of time," he said.

Dr. Panzarella has the time for his five jobs in physical
medicine—from teacher to healer—despite devastating multiple sclerosis. He maintains that lack of interest as well as lack
of time keeps doctors from treating the whole patient. But
though doctors have been trained to treat a disability rather
than the whole person, he sees a change coming. He thinks

medical education is shifting toward treating "the whole man," and that more younger doctors are using this concept in their practices.

"But the old-time doctors, I must admit, either haven't had the training or they're afraid. They shy away from chronic illnesses because they don't know, and they fear their inability to handle the various problems. So they either tell patients to go to a social agency or possibly to a physiatrist such as myself, a medical doctor specializing in rehabilitation medicine. And again, many of the older doctors can only remember physical therapy as a heat, massage, and baking treatment. They're unfamiliar with rehabilitation medicine. They kind of feel that the two are the same, and they're not. This is the reason why most doctors just don't do the whole job that I feel should be done for the patient."

Gerry Shur feels strongly the same way. "How many times does a doctor say, 'Contact the MS Society?' " he asked. "How many times does a doctor notify the society that a new patient needs assistance? A friend of mine learned purely by accident that if he was diagnosed as having MS within a specified number of years after leaving service, VA assumes he contracted it in the service and he's entitled to VA disability benefits. He should not have learned that by accident. I think the doctor should treat the total being with all his problems. The first thing that comes into a guy's mind when he knows he has MS is, 'How will I support my family?' One of the things the doctor can do to alleviate that first concern is to say, 'By the way, I want you to understand that you're entitled to benefits if you've been in the service, or you may be.' [If multiple sclerosis develops to a degree of 10 percent disability within seven years after discharge from the armed forces, the veteran is presumed to have acquired multiple sclerosis in the service and is entitled to veteran's benefits.]

"People know so little about the disease that they think

after an attack they will never go back to work again—if they live. In addition to getting a full explanation from his doctor, a patient in the hospital should be visited by someone who knows from personal experience about the disease. Doctors should arrange that through the MS Society for their patients' peace of mind. It would have made such a difference to me when I had my first attack that I would be willing now to be a hospital visitor myself. I could tell a patient that I have had MS for eleven years and I'm still working full time and more. That's the reassurance I missed."

Rita Dalton's husband recalled an episode last year that he cannot forget. She was hospitalized for doctors to try an electronic device, which it was hoped would stimulate nerve regeneration, and at the same time she was given a brain scan. "When the doctor told me the results," Bill Dalton recalled, "he spoke across her bed just as if she wasn't there. He said there had been no response to the electronic device and the brain scan showed quite a bit of deterioration. Under the circumstances there was no point in even talking about it. All he did was create more emotional problems for her. Either he thought she was not able to understand or it made no difference to him. It made a lot of difference to her—and to me."

If patients become partners with their doctors rather than antagonists, they can move much further along the road to hope.

Jean Ballard discovered that herself as she made the switch from collapsing in tears every time she talked to her doctor (and watching his frustration mount) to calmly reassuring him, "I think I'm going to make it now."

"I was so insecure, so afraid of what was happening that I was constantly asking him, 'Am I going to walk again?' or, 'Am I ever going to be what I was?' I was always asking him the same questions and always on the verge of tears. He didn't think I was emotionally together at all. He didn't think I could cope. At that point, he didn't even use the words MS around me because he thought that made me feel worse."

Then, Jean said, in a group brought together by the local Multiple Sclerosis Society, "I realized that all the doctors were like this because they didn't have the answers. That's why my doctor seemed disgusted with me, and abrupt. He seemed to be acting like 'O God, it's her again' if I called too much when I was frightened by different pains and sensations. In the group, I got a little more together about the disease. When I saw him, instead of asking, 'Am I going to walk again?' I would say, 'It's getting a little easier for me to walk now. What can I do to strengthen my legs to keep this from happening again?' "

As Jean discovered, doctors do not want to get involved in emotional issues because both doctor and patient wind up frustrated. If patients really want a commonsense discussion of their illness, doctors say, they can get it by bringing an agenda to their doctor's appointment and sticking to it. Should she go on a diet and, if so, what kind? Would physiotherapy help strengthen her legs? Must she give up smoking when it is the only vice left? Does vitamin C really prevent colds? Should she take contraceptive pills? Does it injure a teenager's psyche to be given the responsibility for her younger brother when mother has succumbed to a bottomless pit of fatigue? A doctor may not be able to predict how long a patient may be free of attacks or how long a leg will remain stiff, but he can answer specific questions, and those are the answers the patient really wants.

Anne Jackson went through enough misery with doctors to give up all of them if she dared. One doctor told her the problem was a heart condition and her leg dragged because she was having a stroke. She changed doctors and tried to describe the lack of feeling in her arms. "I'd say, 'I know

I'm taking your hand, touching you, but I don't feel it.' He would look at me as if I was a loony bug." While one doctor said she had multiple sclerosis, a second said she did not, and a third said maybe. Neither crybaby nor quitter, Anne was determined to get answers that made sense.

"I wanted finally to deal with a doctor who had the time, patience, and knowledge to tell me the truth," Anne said. "My sister went through *Who's Who in Neurology* to find the right man and I met with him for an hour and a half. I asked him to read my medical record and let me explain my symptoms and then he should ask questions. I told him I knew doctors didn't know everything and I didn't expect him to. I said, 'If you don't know how to deal with my problem, tell me. Don't make any promises. If there's no medication, tell me that, too.' He thanked me for my candor and told me I was the first patient he'd ever met who told him what she wanted from a doctor."

She asked the right questions and got the answers she needed to give a new pattern to her life. Anne has consulted no other doctor since. She believes in him, trusts him, and no one can ask more of a doctor-patient partnership.

For a variety of reasons, patients may give up on doctors. That can be self-defeating, as a Virginia group was told by a physiotherapist: "I know some of you have had bad experiences with doctors, so you don't see a doctor regularly," she told them, "but I'm telling you to keep in touch with your doctor to be sure the rest of your body functions normally."

A pamphlet of the National Multiple Sclerosis Society makes the same point. "Once you give up—once you begin thinking that every ache and pain is related to MS—you greatly increase your chances of ignoring a problem that may have nothing to do with multiple sclerosis. Only your doctor is equipped to pinpoint non-MS-related health hazards, thus saving you a great deal of unnecessary worry."

Diane Afes of the National Capital Chapter of the National Multiple Sclerosis Society worries that patients refuse counseling when they need it. "They'll say, 'They used to think I was going crazy, so I had to go see a shrink.' Then, when they really do have some psychological or emotional problem that goes along with MS, they won't go near a psychiatrist because their initial reaction was so negative. This is really sad because every person with MS should get some kind of support, whether it be from a psychiatrist, psychologist, social worker, or another MS person."

Diane waved at my toppling pile of notebooks full of interviews with my new friends and the stack of taped tales of suffering and hope. "That's why they talked so much to you. Some were lonely, and all this stuff had been building up inside of them. There was a girl the other day, very intelligent but very upset. I told her a lot of things were getting to her and she needed to talk to somebody. She told me, 'I'm not about to go back to them.' "

Donna Matzureff has had the disease for twenty years. She wrote an ode with tears running down her cheeks one day as she felt herself rushing into an exacerbation, yet she is realist enough to understand doctors. There was the doctor who studied her eyes and her records and said, "Christ, what life dishes out!" He never told her what he meant, but Donna commented, "I was very warmed by that because it was honest and compassionate." Later, she was hurt by another doctor who told her in an offhand way as she was leaving the hospital after her worst attack: "You'll have a severe limp but you don't mind that, do you?" She thought him insensitive and cruel. She no longer does, and to a group of young people with multiple sclerosis, she explained why:

"Doctors see people worse off than you and they see you at your worst times, worse off than you are now. If your doctor sees you walking with a cane, he says you're doing fine, but you see yourself as you were playing tennis, dancing, adventuring. And you say, how could he say I'm doing fine when I'm not the way I was. What seems insensitive on his part is not necessarily so. He has a different frame of reference." With the understanding she has now, Donna can forgive.

My own doctor made understanding easy. He told me once that he practiced medicine as though he were the only doctor in the world. He said he had to know enough, stay sufficiently aware of medical advances, to recognize his patients' needs. He knew what I needed because I told him often enough. All I wanted was to keep on working, and he saw to that. When all the patient asks is what is going to happen, the doctor is going to say he does not know and she exits crying, as Jean Ballard used to do. The shopping-list method is ten times as effective. Just as I jot it down when I run out of cereal or celery, I make a note of symptoms and questions: "Pins and needles in my arm when I do sit-ups. Why?" or, "Insomnia. What to take?" or, "Eyelids heavy. MS or need glasses changed?" I telephone his nurse to get the answers for me unless I have to see him, when I pack all my questions into the office visit. It is the efficient way to live with disease.

A doctor who keeps a patient functioning is feeding him hope every day. The first thing that Michael Rubin, the Justice Department attorney, asked his neurologist was, "What can I do and what can't I do?" The doctor replied, "Michael, you can do everything you did before. Just don't fatigue yourself." To this day, Michael told me, he does what he did before but he knows when to stop. Gerry Shur, his colleague, remembered the neurologist telling him: "One thing I could tell you to do is avoid tension, but if you're anything like me, that could create more tension, so go about your life the best you can and enjoy yourself." Gerry Shur is doing just that.

When I embarked on this search for hope, all I heard were

bitter stories about doctors and doctor attitudes that patients described variously as callous, careless, or cowardly. Even some doctors confided that their colleagues shied away from patients they thought were doomed. Until Jonas Salk got involved in the research, only the most dedicated researchers were willing to concentrate on what others considered a lost cause.

Now I have seen for myself that doctors faced with multiple sclerosis are not all the villains I once thought they were. An increasing number are calling and writing the National Institute of Neurological and Communicative Disorders and Stroke at Bethesda, Maryland, to discuss treatment of particular problems, whether certain drugs are past the testing stage, and if there is any truth to rumors of an effective treatment, a cure, or a new diet. At least they care enough now to ask.

Some are doing a lot more than asking. When Dr. Donald Silberberg, head of the Multiple Sclerosis Clinical Research Center at the University of Pennsylvania, discovered that Medicare, Medicaid, and the private insurance companies had stopped paying for injections of ACTH, the corticosteroid used by some physicians to get patients through acute attacks of the disease, he protested to the National Multiple Sclerosis Society and the National Institutes of Health. The trouble had come in March 1977, when the Food and Drug Administration listed all the approved uses for ACTH and omitted multiple sclerosis. In vain the doctors had argued that ACTH helped patients recover from acute attacks. The FDA had followed the finding of a panel organized by the National Academy of Sciences and the National Research Council (both of which are headed by the husband of a multiple sclerosis victim). It was hard to argue with so prestigious a group, but Dr. Silberberg's protests did not go unheeded.

The Neurologic Drugs Advisory Committee, headed by Dr. Guy McKhann, professor of neurology at Johns Hopkins

Medical Institutions, studied evidence amassed by several sources here and abroad and recommended that the FDA approve ACTH for use in acute attacks of the disease. The FDA's Bureau of Drugs still had to approve, but so great was the push to relieve patients of what could be large hospital bills that officials immediately began planning a corner-cutting method of restoring insurers payments for the drug. Anyone who witnessed that effort by leading doctors to save patients money would think again about doctors being indifferent to needs of people with multiple sclerosis.

More doctors now probably would agree with Dr. Tourtellotte when he says: "Almost all MS patients can survive without incapacitating pain and depression, most can be gainfully employed, and many who are talented, skilled, and enthusiastic can create."

Chapter 9

The Detective Story of Research

Shirley Hennesy spent four bitter years trying to find out why she was falling in the street and nearly being run down by cars skidding to avoid her. Even after she broke her arm in a fall down stairs, her doctor was still telling her, "We have to wait." An artist, she had to quit work, give up her ambition to teach art. She was walking with two canes when a National Institute of Neurological and Communicative Disorders and Stroke (NINCDS) researcher told her, "Here's something you can do about multiple sclerosis."

Shirley started helping Dr. Roswell Eldridge, chief of the neurogenetics branch, on his "MS Family Study," getting the "pedigree" of patients with the disease, tracing their families through past generations in search of relatives with the same affliction.

She talks to people throughout the country, prods their memories until they recall an uncle they lost track of who used crutches. Yes, his widow tells them, he had multiple sclerosis.

She feels like a detective tracking down a suspect. And research—even her own insignificant role in it—gives her the same satisfaction she got from art. Her art teacher had once told her that art becomes creation when you do not know how the painting will ultimately look. "It's the same way in research. You don't know what's going to work," she said. "Research is a form of creation because you don't know what you're going to find when you start. I'm still creating—just using different techniques."

The creative process of research is going on all over the world as scientists search for the cause of multiple sclerosis, how to make a positive diagnosis, how to retard or reverse its course, how to prevent or cure it.

The sums being spent on research, particularly in the United States, are climbing steadily under the twin spurs of a hard-hitting report from the congressionally mandated National Advisory Commission on Multiple Sclerosis and ever more promising lines of inquiry. In the United States alone in 1978, more than $38 million was tagged for research, some of it spread over several years. The National Institutes of Health were the largest public source of funding. The National Multiple Sclerosis Society put close to $8.5 million in the research pot and the Kroc Foundation added another million.

Despite increasing funds pouring into research, the disease still defies all efforts to find the cause. Progress comes slowly; research failures still outnumber successes; well-publicized "breakthroughs" fail to prove out and the hopes of patients are crushed so often that they refuse to get excited even when a name as promising as that of Dr. Jonas Salk, who helped conquer polio, is linked to the research.

Yet progress has been made. Dr. Guy McKhann, professor of neurology at Johns Hopkins Medical Institutions, whose own research team has provided some important new information (he shies away from terms like "breakthrough"), contends that the past five years have produced much "that we were not doing or didn't clearly understand before."

While most of the research still centers on trying to find the cause, increasing emphasis is given to finding a surer and speedier method of diagnosis. The McKhann team was seeking ways to positive diagnosis when, instead, it developed a test for identifying the various stages of multiple sclerosis. It is now using that test to get the first objective measure of the efficacy of multiple sclerosis treatment.

The McKhann team test was developed, as so many medical advances are, after an accidental discovery. Dr. Robert Herndon, former director of the Johns Hopkins Hospital Multiple Sclerosis Clinic and now director of the Brain Research Institute at the University of Rochester, was using an electron microscope to observe cerebrospinal fluid from patients with a wide variety of spinal and brain diseases. He was searching for virus particles of another disease when he detected the unmistakable layered cells of myelin fragments in the spinal fluid of a patient who turned out to be in the highly active, acute stage of multiple sclerosis. The fragments had never before been seen in human cerebrospinal fluid.

Using the electron microscope, Johns Hopkins scientists found more bits of myelin in the cerebrospinal fluid of other multiple sclerosis patients. "We decided to look at those bits chemically to see if there was anything unique, anything that stood out, that we could use for a test because doing electron microscopy was cumbersome, difficult, and impractical," Dr. McKhann said.

By now, it was well known that basic protein (BP) is a common component of myelin. In fact, basic protein was being used to produce an experimental disease in animals, about which I will say more later. Dr. McKhann thought it would be possible to make an antibody to BP that could react to minute amounts of it in the spinal fluid.

About that time, Dr. Steven Cohen, working under a postdoctoral fellowship from the National Multiple Sclerosis

Society, joined Dr. McKhann's laboratory. Using guinea pigs and rabbits, he developed a more convenient method for detecting basic protein. The new test is called the basic protein assay, a biochemical test using radioactively labeled antibodies to reveal the presence of specific protein.

With the new radioactive tagging, the McKhann team found evidence of basic protein in the cerebrospinal fluid of many multiple sclerosis patients but seldom in patients with other neurological diseases. Measuring the amount of basic protein in the cerebrospinal fluid, they made an important discovery: In patients in whom the disease is inactive, no myelin basic protein appears in the cerebrospinal fluid; in patients who have a slowly progressing form of the disease, low levels of BP appear; but patients experiencing an acute attack show high levels of BP.

"We can now measure when an acute attack is subsiding," Dr. McKhann said, "because the BP level begins to fall back toward normal. With this test, we are developing a much more exact way of observing the course of the disease, which in turn should enable us to assess the effectiveness of drug therapy more exactly."

That in itself is an important advance because until now there has been no way to measure objectively whether the drugs patients take to subdue an attack actually do any good. "By using the BP assay," McKhann said, "we are able to start and stop therapy more wisely because we can tell when an attack is subsiding and when it is not."

McKhann considers his test, now being used at Johns Hopkins and at two other centers that treat many multiple sclerosis patients, still very much at the investigative stage. "It's new information which we hope will be useful to us in evaluation of patients. It will be at least another year before we know how valuable this test will be." He does not want it to be set up all over the country yet because he wants to be sure it is set up right. "It will gradually be done in more centers, but I don't think we are ready to put this in every hospital that wants to look at the spinal fluid of MS patients until we are absolutely sure of all the parameters—where one can get in trouble doing the test, how one interprets it."

Dr. McKhann is looking for a way to use more accessible blood or urine rather than tapping of patients' spinal fluid. He is hoping that a component of broken-down myelin other than BP may be easier to find in the blood and urine.

Meanwhile, he has not forgotten his original hope that the finding of BP in cerebrospinal fluid could lead to a diagnostic test. He hopes it can meet one critical problem in trying to pin down a multiple sclerosis diagnosis. That problem is the first attack.

"We now make a diagnosis," Dr. McKhann said, "by looking for repeated episodes in different parts of the nervous system. If a patient comes in with an acute attack involving only one part of the nervous system, we have neither of our two clinical criteria [different symptoms, different times]. So it would be helpful to see the reaction to the BP test."

When a patient comes in with no previous history of multiple sclerosis, "we are not able to say yet that finding BP in the spinal fluid means he has the disease. We just don't have that data." To get the data, the McKhann group will test the spinal fluid of forty patients who may be having a first attack of multiple sclerosis and following their medical history for a period of time to determine whether they turn out to have multiple sclerosis or not. Thus it may take several years to learn if they are on the right track. Such is the slow pace of multiple sclerosis research.

As often happens in medical research, despite the years of checking and cross-checking results, two research teams can arrive at the same answers at almost the same time. Thus, while the McKhann group in Baltimore was developing a radioimmunoassay to measure BP in the cerebrospinal fluid, Dr. John Whitaker of the Veterans Administration Hospital in Memphis, Tennessee, was using goats to perfect a similar test, called a double antibody radioimmunoassay, in his neurology laboratory. His goal also was to reach an objective and reliable evaluation of the multiple sclerosis process and to evaluate the effects of treatment.

Although Dr. Whitaker and the McKhann group worked entirely independently of each other, their goals were similar. Dr. McKhann said the primary difference between the two tests was in interpretation of the nature of the material observed in the spinal fluid. "Our impression is that it's been the whole basic protein molecule and Dr. Whitaker thinks it's fragments of it, that the molecule has been chewed up a little bit before it gets there. But that's the only difference."

Patients are deeply interested in what causes multiple sclerosis and in possible methods of treatment but their first concern is diagnosis. And with reason. The four years that Shirley Hennesy waited to find out what she had was not unusual in the 1960s. There is still no established laboratory test that is a specific diagnostic test for multiple sclerosis. To be of any value, the test has to be able to do more than distinguish patients with multiple sclerosis from well persons. It must be able to distinguish them from patients with any other neurological disease. And that is where most tests break down, where overlap occurs, where patients with some other diseases react to the test in the same way as those with multiple sclerosis.

Three newly refined tests of the cerebrospinal fluid can aid diagnosis—aid, but not carry the diagnosis alone. As always, physicians are told to use the new tests in concert with the old different-times-and-places clinical diagnosis. Although still not the long-sought test to pin down multiple sclerosis as definitely as a biopsy reveals the presence of cancer, these tests are more refined and revealing than earlier tests. Since the tests can be done routinely in any diagnostic laboratory, the doctor no longer has to send the patient's spinal fluid to some specialized center.

All three tests relate to IgG irregularities in cerebrospinal fluid. IgG is a class of proteins containing antibodies that the body makes in defense against substances the body considers alien to it. The test considered most convenient and most likely to reveal abnormalities detects the presence of oligoclonal immunoglobulin G (IgG) bands. Dr. Kenneth P. Johnson, head of the Multiple Sclerosis Clinical Research Center at the University of California, San Francisco, and chief of the Neurology Research Laboratory at the San Francisco Veterans Administration Hospital, says that cerebrospinal fluid, concentrated fifty times, will produce readily apparent bands in the fluid of multiple sclerosis patients. Studies performed in Europe and confirmed in this country show such bands in approximately 90 percent of patients with definite multiple sclerosis.

By means of a laboratory technique, electrophoresis, Dr. Johnson has been comparing patterns of IgG bands in the spinal fluid of multiple sclerosis patients and those with other central nervous system diseases in hopes of improving the bands' diagnostic usefulness.

Another new method seeks to aid diagnosis from a single neurological symptom occurring anywhere in the central nervous system. The doctor may request electrophysiologic measurements of the visual system, even if there is no eye problem at the time. Since eyes are so frequently involved in multiple sclerosis damage, it is a likely place to look for an early clue.

If the measurement shows visual system abnormalities, the doctor can suspect a disease occurring in many locations like multiple sclerosis. These new measurements to get what is called evoked potential response may solve the long-perplexing problem of diagnosis when only a single ailment is present. The method is now being widely and routinely used.

Help with difficult multiple sclerosis diagnosis is now available from scientists at any of the seven NINCDS-supported clinical research centers set up in recent years to study multiple sclerosis. NINCDS can supply both the name of the nearest center and a summary of current research.

The time lag between onset of the disease and firm diagnosis vexes researchers as it does patients. The delay in diagnosis is considered a serious deterrent to research as it tends to focus on the disease at a time remote from its onset, and this interval of time may cause research to focus on elements in the aftermath of the disease process rather than the genesis of the disease itself.

Since 1962, studies indirectly relating the measles virus and other viruses to multiple sclerosis have yielded similar results —no proof. What looked briefly like a breakthrough, a way to pin measles to multiple sclerosis, came in 1976 when doctors at Long Island College Hospital and Kings County Hospital reported finding measles antigen in the small bowel of thirty patients with multiple sclerosis but none in a control group of patients without multiple sclerosis. (Antigens are substances that stimulate an "immune response.") The scientists theorized that chronic measles infection persisted in the small bowel. The possibility was provocative, but so far scientists in other laboratories have failed to confirm it.

The search for a multiple sclerosis virus has been challenging scientists for years. Evidence from the laboratory that a virus was present in multiple sclerosis victims was obtained in 1972 from Richard I. Carp and his colleagues at the New York State Institute for Basic Research in Mental Retardation on Staten Island. They inoculated mice with extracts of brain, blood, and tissue from victims and found that there was a sharp drop in the blood count of a type of white cell known as polymorphonuclear leukocyte. No such change occurred after tissues from patients with other disorders were injected into the mice. In addition, brain extracts and serum from mice previously inoculated with multiple sclerosis material caused a white-cell drop when given to other mice, suggesting that whatever was in the multiple sclerosis patients' tissues grew and multiplied just as a virus would be expected to do.

For the next four years, the Carp findings were met with considerable skepticism largely because white-cell counts in mice are highly variable and no one was able to repeat the original experiments with the same results. In December of 1975, however, two husband-wife research teams in Philadelphia not only confirmed the Carp theory but added to it. Although many scientists continued to doubt the validity of the observations because the assay systems employed were so complex, the research was widely hailed in the press, particularly after *Lancet,* the noted British medical journal,* editorialized that the American findings placed multiple sclerosis "squarely in the sector of infectious diseases, although the precise nature of the virus has yet to be determined." My own newspaper, *The Washington Star,* noting that *Lancet* said the American findings seem to remove multiple sclerosis from the list of diseases of unknown cause, headlined the story: "Multiple Sclerosis Break-Through?" Within eighteen months, the question mark was justified. First, the Staten Island and Philadelphia researchers both termed premature the *Lancet* conclusion that a viral cause of the disease had been found. The hopes of patients, of their doctors, and other scientists were finally knocked out in October 1977, when the Philadelphia investigators joined the Staten Island team in questioning the validity of their own earlier observations and in concluding

* "A Milestone in Multiple Sclerosis," *The Lancet,* Feb. 28, 1976, pp. 459–460.

that the assay system used should be discontinued as too complex.

Another test, the "rosette" blood test for multiple sclerosis, got a premature ride in the press simply because the prospect of a way to test for multiple sclerosis that did not involve being stabbed in the spine sounded so promising. Dr. Nelson L. Levy, Paul S. Auerbach, and Dr. Edward C. Hayes in the Division of Immunology at the Duke University Medical Center attracted national attention after reporting in the June 1976 issue of the *New England Journal of Medicine* that they had a blood test that showed potential for practical diagnosis of the baffling disease. Levy said tests that Auerbach, a third-year medical student, was conducting as part of his training actually led to the test's development.

The new blood test, said Dr. Levy in his 1976 report, is accurate, can distinguish between multiple sclerosis and certain other neurological diseases, and can indicate multiple sclerosis regardless of the severity, duration, and activity of the disease. The blood test mixed a person's white cells with tissue culture cells infected with measles virus. This resulted in formation of clumps, called rosettes, of white cells in patterns around the virus-infected tissue culture cells.

For the test, twenty-seven patients with multiple sclerosis were compared with twenty-six patients with varied neurological problems and with ten healthy persons from the laboratory and clinical staff at the Duke University Medical Center. More patients were tested later.

The researchers found more rosettes and often larger ones in the multiple sclerosis patients than in healthy persons and those with other diseases. The difference was so marked, with no overlap, that it indicated "the diagnostic potential of the rosetting phenomenon."

Enthusiasm generated by the report was tempered by an editorial by Dr. Martin S. Hirsch of Massachusetts General

Hospital warning that "several reservations must be kept in mind before the authors' conclusions are accepted too readily." One reservation was the need for testing a wider range of patients free of multiple sclerosis but suffering from other conditions, including viral diseases and disorders of the immune system. Two years later, Levy and the Duke group still had not proved the value of the method as a specific and practical diagnostic test. The test required tissue infected with measles virus, but when the researcher started to ship the target cells, they could not survive freezing. Dr. Levy still hopes to confirm the specificity of the test and to find a way for it to be more useful.

In multiple sclerosis research the pace may be slow but it is steadily forward and periodically punctuated with advances. Typical is the tadpole test. A tadpole with a transparent optic nerve is providing a new and direct look at the destruction of the myelin nerve covering by cerebrospinal fluid from multiple sclerosis patients.

In effect, this test becomes a show window for what happens to humans because of demyelination—the patchy destruction of the myelin sheath around the nerve fibers of the central nervous system. The tadpole model represents the first time a living system has been used to observe demyelinating activity.

Initial studies of the tadpole involved forty-six patients, including some with multiple sclerosis, some with a disorder of the optic nerve, and patients with other neurological disorders.

Dr. Henry Webster and his colleagues at NINCDS, who developed the tadpole model, found that cerebrospinal fluid from multiple sclerosis patients injected into tissue surrounding the tadpole's optic nerve diffuses quickly and penetrates the optic nerve. Researchers with a special microscope can then actually count the resulting myelin lesions, which in humans bare the nerve fibers and cause impulses from the brain to go astray.

The reaction of the tadpole's optic nerve is additionally interesting to researchers because the optic nerve in humans is frequently effected early in the course of multiple sclerosis, producing temporary "blind spots" in the center of vision—what I used to describe as my "jigsaw-puzzle" vision.

The scientists eyeing the tadpole examined peripheral nerves near the optic nerve and made what may be a significant observation. The peripheral nerves were not demyelinated by the cerebrospinal fluid. That suggests that whatever causes myelin destruction is aimed specifically against myelin in the central nervous system—the brain and spinal cord.

Scientists discovered that the toxic agent in the spinal fluid appears shortly after an active attack of multiple sclerosis, suggesting that it may even produce the attack. In terms of the number of lesions, the toxic agent does its worst damage two days after infection and becomes less destructive later, indicating that lesions are reversible and that damaged areas could recover.

One great thing about the tadpole test is how economical it is with spinal fluid. Other demyelination studies on tissue culture by various scientists around the world required a concentrated "pool" of fluid from many patients before demyelination could be observed. Only one-sixtieth of an ounce of cerebrospinal fluid was needed for the tadpole test.

The tadpole-test results opened up all manner of possibilities for further study but also produced one negative. Researchers found the test may not be useful for diagnosis because fluid from participants with "possible MS" did not cause demyelination. A year later, when the disease had progressed, fluid taken from one participant did cause demyelination then.

Some of the most promising research on cause is exploring the peculiar immune response of persons with multiple sclerosis—how their bodies react both to outside "invaders" and to substances of self which they mistake for invaders.

Researchers say there is no question that the immune system, the body's defense system, is involved one way or another in multiple sclerosis. The challenge prompting immunological research to mushroom is to find out how the immune system is involved. Whether the fault is too much immunity or too little or some other defect, there's no question but that something is definitely wrong with the immune system. "Just knowing that," said one researcher, "gives us a real lead."

Dr. McKhann said that all the work under way on viruses and immunoglobulin G (gamma globulin) strongly suggests that multiple sclerosis patients have a peculiar hyperimmune state in which antibodies are being produced locally in the brain by cells that are not normal residents of brain tissue. "So there is something very peculiar about the immunological state of these patients. That is definite knowledge which is now sorting itself out. It's reflected in antibodies to specific components such as viruses, the increased gamma globulins, the bands in the cerebrospinal fluid."

The finding of the increased IgG in the cerebral spinal fluid was the first indication that people with multiple sclerosis may have an immune response different from healthy people's. The second indication is the different level of antibodies to a range of viruses they have either in the blood or spinal fluid. Measles is the most widely studied one. It is not a massive difference, scientists say, but a consistent one. Patients, their brothers and sisters and close relatives without the disease, also tend to have a higher level of measles antibodies than other people without multiple sclerosis. That still does not mean measles has anything to do with multiple sclerosis. Patients with MS have antibodies to other viruses besides measles.

Once investigators have concluded that persons with multiple sclerosis have different immune responses from other people's and that some of this difference is shared by close relatives, the next step is to find whether some association exists between susceptibility to the disease and inherited characteristics.

Body cell types such as the red blood cell types important in transfusions or the white blood cell types now important in organ transplant work are inherited. If the types of donor and receiver fail to match when doctors try to transplant an organ, the immune system will rise up and destroy the transplant. The immune system has the ability to recognize the difference between self and foreign substances. These include tissue types that are inherited from the genes of father and mother and "unique" in the selection of genes in each individual. The only exceptions are identical twins, who share the same pattern of cell types. Certain of these cell types occur more often in MS patients than in other people. In basic studies of animals, it has now been demonstrated that the genes which control tissue types are closely related to the regulating of immunity.

Since the patterns of immune response that patients with multiple sclerosis inherit from their parents differ generally from that of people who do not have the disease, some investigators believe that there *is* an inherited susceptibility to multiple sclerosis. Researchers do not believe multiple sclerosis itself is inherited, but there is now evidence that susceptibility may be.

Dr. McKhann, for one, thinks a "genetic predisposition" is too strong a term. "I don't want people of a certain lymphocyte [white blood cell] type to feel they are greatly at risk of getting MS," he said. "I don't think we can say that, because for every person with a particular lymphocyte type who gets MS there are probably a thousand who don't, so I'm not sure what word is best. Clearly, there's a finding that's holding up, that if you're of a particular genetic makeup, the chance of getting MS is higher than if you don't have that makeup. That's where things stand now."

Dr. William E. Reynolds, deputy director of the National MS Society's research programs, stresses that if a person inherits a particular genetic pattern, presumably he risks getting multiple sclerosis if he encounters something in the environment that might trigger it. "Another person," he said, "may be exposed to the same things in the environment—virus or whatever—and if his immune system is different, he's not going to get MS."

Both mice and men literally are involved in the efforts of NINCDS to pin down the association with inherited cell types. In the Neuroimmunological Branch, Drs. Dale E. McFarlin, chief, and Henry F. McFarland, assistant chief, are studying virus-induced central nervous system diseases in strains of selectively inbred mice. Paralleling the laboratory studies are the studies of families in which more than one member has the disease. It was one of those studies that used the volunteer services of Shirley Hennesy. One study involves identical and nonidentical twins. Only identical twins share immune system genes; thus, for nonidentical twins as well as relatives and strangers, these genes are the mark of biologic individuality.

A massive study is proceeding in the Scottish Orkney and Shetland islands, scene of the highest known prevalence of multiple sclerosis in the world. There, 250 persons out of every 100,000 are victims. Elsewhere, the rate may vary from 20 or less in low-risk areas in the southern temperate zone to 80 per 100,000 in more northerly high-risk areas.

The islands are a valuable setting for investigators not only because of the high rate but because the islands pride themselves on keeping extraordinarily good records of parish marriages and death certificates. Investigators can trace back genetic lineage two hundred years. They try to find out whether the incidence can be tracked to a particular family, as was true of another neurological disorder, Huntington's disease, in the United States.

A third angle of the attack is a study of viruses and the immune system of 100 regularly followed patients at the NINCDS-sponsored Multiple Sclerosis Clinical Research Center at the University of Pennsylvania in collaboration with the Wistar Institute of Anatomy and Biology. A fourth study, by a NINCDS grantee at UCLA, follows 150 families with at least 2 members with the illness, including 75 families with close relatives stricken. Of particular interest is a cluster of patients in King County, Washington, where 8 students in the same high school graduating class of 1953 now have multiple sclerosis. They are typical of several clusters of patients reported in various high-risk areas around the country.

Since investigators agree that the inherited immune system is involved one way or another, they are investigating the possibility that the body's defense against outside invaders like viruses can also turn against self as has been established in such other diseases as myasthenia gravis and lupus erythematosus.

The possibility that multiple sclerosis is an autoimmune disease—the body attacking itself—has been studied for years in an experimental disease known as experimental allergic encephalomyelitis (EAE). This is the experimental disease on which many scientists have been working.

Researchers have long been hampered by the fact that multiple sclerosis has no counterpart in animals. To compensate for that, researchers developed EAE, which can be induced in animals using myelin basic protein taken from central nervous system tissue material. EAE in animals produces demyelination and scar tissue similar to multiple sclerosis in man. It had been regarded as an imperfect model for multiple sclerosis because it had no exacerbating-remitting course. That objection was removed when three groups of investigators produced chronic and relapsing forms of the model disease. Experiments with the model have told investigators much about regulating and controlling the immune system, but a direct relationship between multiple sclerosis and EAE has not been established.

One key difference between the two diseases is that multiple sclerosis patients do not have any, or have only a very low level, of antibodies—the body's defense weapon—to basic protein, as animals do with EAE. The possibility exists, though, that since the model disease can be seen at a much earlier stage than multiple sclerosis is ever seen by a doctor, a person also might have these antibodies early in the disease, although years later, when the patient is first examined, the antibodies might be tied up somewhere else, maybe in the brain. In other words, the model disease superficially may not match multiple sclerosis because our timing is off. The human patient cannot be studied at the same time in the course of the disease as the animal.

Incidentally, the animal can be treated and can recover from the experimental disease by use of a variation of the same material that made him sick.

Like many other investigators, Dr. Jonas Salk has been concerned with experiments with EAE for ten years; for the past five years he has conducted a large number of experiments in guinea pigs to determine what kind of basic proteins work best and how much to give to treat the disease.

The interest of Eli Lilly, an Indianapolis-based drug company, was aroused because there had never been commercial production of basic protein. The Food and Drug Administration has now approved a Lilly preparation of myelin basic protein as an investigational new drug. Until now, laboratories have simply made up a batch as they needed it for experiments. Many laboratories had been using cows because cow brain was readily available from any slaughterhouse. Pigs were chosen over cows for the basic protein in the Salk experiments and the Lilly drug because pigs are a source of insulin in humans and much is known about human reaction to material from pigs.

Neither Dr. Salk nor the drug company was responsible for the sudden flood of publicity about Dr. Salk's intention to make human tests to see if an allergic reaction causes multiple sclerosis following the theory of the body being allergic to itself. It all began on a mid-January weekend in 1978 when a television reporter in Indianapolis stumbled on what he considered a "scoop" and nobody could talk him out of it by telling him his story was premature.

By Monday, the wire services had picked it up; by Tuesday, radio commentators had stripped the story to a bald, misleading announcement that Dr. Salk had approval from the Food and Drug Administration to test a vaccine for multiple sclerosis; by midweek Dr. Salk had to put on more staff simply to deal with inquiries.

To quiet the furor, Dr. Salk put out a brief statement, saying multiple sclerosis is a disease of unknown cause, that there are many theories, none of which has yet been substantiated. "One theory is that MS is an autoallergic disease," Dr. Salk went on in the statement. "This means that the immune system reacts as if there was an allergy to specific components in brain and spinal cord. However, even if MS were an auto-allergic disease then the causative substance still remains to be established.

"For many years, an experimental autoallergic disease called experimental allergic encephalomyelitis (EAE) has been studied in animals. Its cause is known to be an allergic reaction to a specific protein in brain and spinal cord. Investigations are soon to be undertaken in patients with MS to determine whether it is due to a similar allergic reaction.

"The study to be carried out in patients will require several years before conclusions can be drawn as to its significance in clarifying the cause of MS."

He makes no suggestion that the experiments, closely supervised by the FDA, could lead to successful treatment of multiple sclerosis in humans as it does with EAE in animals and, in fact, earlier attempts to treat European patients this way were unsuccessful. But the first handful of patients must have contemplated at least progress toward treatment as they volunteered for Salk tests that could take years to be successful or fail in months.

Science still cannot offer a treatment to arrest the progress of the disease or reverse its course, although several approaches remain under study. Some scientists are trying to increase the immune response of multiple sclerosis patients. The immuno-reactive drug levamisole is being tested in twenty-five multiple sclerosis patients at the NINCDS-supported Multiple Sclerosis Clinical Research Center at Emory University, as well as at the Belgium National Center for Multiple Sclerosis at Mels-broek.

Several methods of ameliorating symptoms are being tested. One is the experimental use of Chlorpromazine and Dilantin in combination to suppress spasticity. One patient in tests at

Georgetown University in Washington, D.C., tells friends a before-and-after story. She was so stiff that her husband had to bend her legs for her before he left for work in the morning so she could sit in her wheelchair. The combined medication, she says, has relieved that terrible stiffness.

Scientists at the UCLA Clinical Research Center are using two drugs, methyl-dopa and dibenzyline, for relief of bladder spasticity, which causes incontinence. The drugs' action on bladder sphincters relieves urinary urgency. In one of the most important advances in treatment to date, an investigator at Albert Einstein College of Medicine reported adapting a surgical technique, making an incision in the bladder that is kept closed except when the patient inserts a catheter to void four times daily. Work is continuing on possible development of electrical stimulation to provide bladder control.

Medical history teaches that diseases can be successfully treated or prevented before their cause is established, but the lion's share of research money, both government and private, still goes to trying to find the cause of multiple sclerosis.

The best evidence so far that multiple sclerosis may result from contact with something in the environment during childhood or adolescence comes from studies of geography and migration. Years ago, when I worked on murder stories, detectives would tell me that the first step toward solving the crime was getting the right questions to ask. Scientists trying to solve the crime of multiple sclerosis are finding the right questions to ask. What helps them is the post–World War II science of geographic medicine. If they know where in the world the disease strikes most often, they are ready to ask: Why there? What is true of that environment that is not true somewhere else? What way of life, what diet, what climate seems to encourage multiple sclerosis, possibly triggering a latent virus to show itself?

Close to two hundred studies around the world have provided scientists some idea of where multiple sclerosis crops up most often or is virtually unknown. Multiple sclerosis becomes more prevalent in the temperate zone the farther you get from the equator. Thus, the disease appears more frequently in northern Germany than southern Italy, more often in New England than the Southwest, much more often on both sides of the Canadian border than the Mexican border.

The dividing line between high-risk northern United States and medium-risk southern states appears to be at the Mason-Dixon line, just about Washington, D.C. In Europe, the disease shows itself across a band of risk greatest in the Orkney and Shetland islands, encompasses Great Britain, and moves across southerly Scandinavia. In the Southern Hemisphere, south Australia, Tasmania, and New Zealand are all rated high-risk areas. Studies are yet to be made in South America.

Geographic medicine has provided other clues that remind some, but not all, researchers of what they discovered about polio. In Hawaii, more Caucasians get multiple sclerosis than Asiatics. It does not strike heavily in the Orient or in most of Africa. A South African study failed to turn up a single case in its sizable Bantu population as of the 1960s and only two since then, but for English-speaking whites, South Africa was an area of medium risk. Even in the United States, multiple sclerosis appears so much oftener among whites than blacks that one researcher quipped: "MS is the white man's burden." Some of my friends with multiple sclerosis in predominantly black Washington, D.C., are black, but most of them came from the North rather than the South. In the United States, the risk of MS among blacks is less than half that of whites, Dr. Kurtzke said a study shows.

The ethnic differences prompted some researchers to make an analogy with polio. When scientists were trying to figure out why Orientals escaped crippling polio, it finally became evident that the health habits of the Orientals, particularly the way they fertilized their vegetables with human excrement, gave infants a mild form of the disease without crippling them and built up an immunity that spared them from getting the paralyzing polio of later years.

Some researchers theorize the same pattern might apply to multiple sclerosis. The hygiene of the Bantus, for instance, is much more primitive than the health habits of the South African whites, so the Bantus may be building up an immunity that the whites lack. In the same way, the Dutch-speaking Afrikaners brought up by Bantu nurses develop the disease far less often than do Europeans who migrate to South Africa.

At what age the Europeans migrate, however, makes a major difference. Dr. Geoffrey Dean of the Medico-Social Research Board of Ireland found that among migrants to South Africa from northern and central Europe the disease occurred in about 49 of each 100,000 people, compared with 11 of each 100,000 English-speaking native South Africans and 3 per 100,000 Afrikaners. What emerged as the key finding was that if Europeans came to South Africa before they were fifteen, they took on the lower risk of the native-born.

The age of fifteen also appeared crucial in the study in Israel made by Dr. Milton Alter of Temple University School of Medicine. Dr. Alter, like Dr. Dean in South Africa, determined that the immigrants to Israel from northern Europe—often from high-risk Russia—retained the risk of their homeland if they came to Israel after they were fifteen. Dr. Alter found a different twist, though. He discovered that children of Afro-Asian immigrants to Israel took on a higher multiple sclerosis rate than their parents.

In searching for clues, medical investigators will hit upon communities with a multiple sclerosis puzzle. In Lewis County, Washington, they discovered that 7 people who had lived in the village of Mossybank, population 415, developed multiple sclerosis. All but one of them shared the disease with a brother, sister, or cousin and all but the same one had had smallpox during a 1924 epidemic. Curiously, Lewis County showed no deaths from smallpox in that epidemic, but during the first half of 1924, 13 deaths were attributed to measles. Since measles—or a complication of measles—is mentioned in speculation about a multiple sclerosis virus, finding those measles deaths gave investigators one more puzzle to ponder.

Clusters of cases crop up periodically in the high-risk northern United States to precipitate searches for what in the environment there might have been the culprit. In one small Massachusetts community, investigators discovered that during the years when a number of young people who developed multiple sclerosis had lived in that town there was widespread contamination of sewage in the water supply. More clues but no answers there or in King County, Washington, where eight members of the same 1953 high school graduating class later developed multiple sclerosis—the cluster now being studied. I found my own cluster of multiple sclerosis victims. Penny Renzi told me that three members of her wedding party later developed the illness—Penny, the bride; her matron of honor; and her bridesmaid. All three had grown up in Massachusetts.

When investigators link where persons with multiple sclerosis live with how they live, the polio pattern could be significant. As Dr. Kurtzke discovered with his continuing survey of World War II veterans, the men who developed multiple sclerosis on the average came from middle-class or affluent homes, scored higher on army intelligence tests and were better educated on the average than the matched controls. Their higher standard of living, as with the victims of polio, could be their curse. At least, that's where the polio comparison takes some investigators.

Age could be another point of comparison. It is generally

accepted now that when polio strikes in infancy, it usually brings lifelong immunity without paralysis, but when it strikes later, it cripples—or crippled, until the Salk vaccine came along. Investigators of multiple sclerosis have reason to believe that the age when a child gets the measles could be relevant here. In the tropics, measles comes earlier than it does in the temperate zone, where the risk of multiple sclerosis increases. In Nigeria or Guatemala, for instance, investigators found almost everyone had had measles before the age of five, while in England and the northern United States, people didn't develop their measles immunity usually until they were six to eight years old. Investigators also discovered that in Finland the victims of multiple sclerosis had usually had measles later than their friends. Researchers haven't yet found a causative link between measles and multiple sclerosis, but in two diseases believed to be a delayed reaction to measles infection the age at which the patient had measles is a relevant factor.

As the studies of South African and Israeli immigrants demonstrated, the age of fifteen seems to be critical. However, there are conflicting explanations of what it means. Dr. Dean believes that a childhood infection without crippling, as in polio, provides later immunity from multiple sclerosis and that such an infection is very common in such low-risk regions as South Africa. On the other hand, Dr. Kurtzke believes the disease is "caught" at about the age of fifteen in high-risk regions like northern Europe but doesn't show itself for years later, regardless of where the person lives.

Both concepts fit the theory that multiple sclerosis is caused by something in the environment, possibly a "slow virus" that remains in the body for many years before the first outward sign. Speculation but no proof exists that the slow virus may be a mutation of measles. The basic difference between the Kurtzke and Dean theories is whether investigators should look for the cause in a low-risk area, where it strikes without lasting effect in childhood and grants lifelong immunity as with polio, or in high-risk areas, where it strikes later and harmfully. "To define which of these is correct," said Dr. Kurtzke, "could well give us the answer to what indeed is this disease we call multiple sclerosis."

The answer may not be too far away now and that, too, could become part of the polio analogy. The kinship between those combating polio and multiple sclerosis goes back to the 1940s when Basil O'Connor, the knowledgeable chairman of the National Foundation for Infantile Paralysis, helped the young Sylvia Lawry found the National Multiple Sclerosis Society.

Many years later, after Dr. Salk discovered the polio vaccine, the National Multiple Sclerosis Society enlisted his expertise. His contribution goes beyond his present work at the Salk Institute in San Diego. As national multiple sclerosis board members freely admit, until Dr. Salk found the way to conquer polio the society had trouble interesting investigators in doing neurological research at all because they could see no hopeful results. These days, leading scientists are going into multiple sclerosis research. "We are engaged in basic research aimed at piecing together the puzzle of multiple sclerosis," Dr. Salk has said repeatedly, "and I believe its time has come."

A quarter century ago, only the most optimistic would have believed polio could be conquered. Now optimists like Dr. Salk believe multiple sclerosis could be next. Certainly, more has been learned about the disease in the decade of the 1970s than in the previous century. Multiple sclerosis researchers may not have the answers, but they now have the right questions—and that is a giant step on the road to hope.

To Dr. Kurtzke, viewing progress as both a leading neurologist treating patients and a researcher seeking clues the world over, the most hopeful thing out of research so far is that multiple sclerosis is indeed a much more benign illness than most people had thought. Secondly, he said, with an epidemiological approach, "we might be able to pin down what this disease is all about." It's likely that once a specific cause is known, a specific treatment will follow. Most patients, he feels, even advanced patients, could profit from effective treatment because "the permanent destruction of tissue" is less common than had been imagined.

Dr. Reynolds was equally emphatic that there is no destruction of the nerve fiber. The nerve cell body is intact; only the myelin is destroyed—selectively destroyed. As Dr. Reynolds put it to me: "The nerve fiber is alive and well, except for the loss of its myelin sheath." That implies that if an MS patient keeps his muscles tuned up, he will be in a better position to benefit from effective treatment when it comes.

Chapter 10

God's Help, Self-Help, and Helping Others

Twenty-nine and pregnant with her seventh child, Alma Gaghan was told she had multiple sclerosis. She spent the night crying and playing solitaire. In the morning, she went to mass and came away convinced that the Lord would not put on her shoulders more of a burden than she could carry. Believing, she carried it through years of diapers and dishes and helping her husband Jim in his contracting business. In 1978, she lost Jim to a heart attack. At the time, I told her to take it easy, that the shock of sudden death could worsen her illness, but she was too busy running her husband's business to heed warnings. She wound up in the hospital.

As soon as she was able to walk, she did what she had always done in a crisis. She talked to God. She told Him she wanted to save her husband's business for their sons. "If it's not Your will to keep on with the business," she added, "I will give it up but please give me a sign." The next day, a call came from a former associate of her husband's. If she wished, he would come back to help with the business. She had her answer.

When Loretta W. Brown went into the hospital with a multiple sclerosis attack in June 1977, paralysis had struck her gag reflex. Instead of food going down to her stomach, it went into her lungs. Even a sip of water could suffocate her. Her arms were paralyzed and she was seeing double. The second night, she stopped breathing. She roused to find people all around her begging her to open her eyes. She gave them a sleepy smile and went back to sleep. Then the tubes began— a tube down her throat to feed her, a tube to supply oxygen, a tube to help her breathe. After weeks, she begged them to remove the tube down her throat because it had become so sore she was sure her gag reflex would never come back until her throat healed. Now, they fed her intravenously, but after a week or ten days, the veins collapsed. The surgeons proposed to insert a tube in her stomach to feed her.

Would that be the only operation or would there be spin-off operations? She had sung classical music. Would a tracheotomy follow the other operation and end her singing? She decided her faith in God was strong enough to put her among the one in five or six who recovered their gag reflex naturally. She refused to allow the operation.

The doctors warned her if she refused surgery, she could not live. If she put anything in her mouth, it would get in her lungs and that would be the end. She still insisted, and her neurologist and internist backed her. For five days, she lived on crushed ice—her own idea. It melted so slowly it was only a trickle down her throat, not enough to choke her. At the end of five days, she knew she had won. Her throat, freed from the tube's irritation, had healed. Her faith had triumphed over even the most modern medicine.

Eliza Ann Dobson had run an elevator in Internal Revenue Service headquarters for many years before her frequent falls led to a diagnosis of multiple sclerosis. With nobody to take care of her, she had been sent to a city-owned convalescent hospital. She was in a wheelchair months later when she finished "Fret Not." She sang her spiritual into a tape recorder and a friendly pastor scored it for her.

From the first, she knew what she would do with her song. She would sell it at a dollar a sheet to raise money for multiple sclerosis research because she was so grateful to the local Multiple Sclerosis Society for parties, her wheelchair, and a feeling "they really care for me." Her impulse, however, to turn over the $500 she made on the song to the society had a deeper root. She had lived to fifty-one before multiple sclerosis stopped her. Young people with the illness had not been so fortunate. They would never have a life, she said, unless research finds a cure. For them, she wrote in her spiritual, "Some day, somewhere, everything is sweet and fair. No more pain and misery. . . ."

These women share something beyond their illness. Each has a working faith, a determination to survive on her own terms, and an encompassing desire to help others. I am convinced those three ingredients can heal when no medicine can —at least no drug or shot or pill science has yet found.

This is no Pollyanna prescription. These women and scores of other women and men I have met turn their backs on instant cures or the persuasions of itinerant faith healers. They expect no miracles but they do believe that the Lord helps those who help themselves—and others.

For those who believe or come to believe in prayer, a form of spiritual healing follows. Expecting no cure they find the next best thing—a life of activity and acceptance.

Bess Maloy had been an athlete—swam on the swimming team, played hockey and basketball, took the lead in the dance pageant at Oberlin College. At twenty-four she felt she was falling apart. None of the doctors she saw for separate ailments put it together, even after she read a magazine article about multiple sclerosis and asked the latest doctor if that was what she had. He told her to forget it and go to a party that night. At the party she collapsed.

For months she spent most of her time in bed. She hid her

sleeping pills, figuring that if she became too much of a burden on her husband and children she would find her own
solution. Then, she too tried prayer. She said if God wanted
her to raise her three children, she would manage somehow.
Her husband could not raise them alone. She crawled up to
the attic and dug out her old maternity corset. Her doctor
warned that she would get dependent on it, but she paid no
attention. She figured that if she could stay up longer with the
corset on, she could exercise and even get to the pool to swim
her way back to health.

With the children she summered by a Michigan lake and
encountered a more active religion. Her landlady's grandfather, a medical missionary, had left books on spiritual healing. She could only read three lines at a time at first because
of her eyes but she covered her good eye to force her bad
eye to work and read on. By the end of the summer, swimming was strengthening her legs and she could even bicycle.
"The physical exercise was important," Bess Maloy says now,
"but more important was the change in my way of thinking.
I realized my mental and emotional attitudes weren't healthy
and needed to be changed. I couldn't change them. The only
one who could was the Lord."

She began buying religious records to play as she ironed,
cooked, and cleaned.

"I was getting all these positive thoughts that God can heal
and does heal. I should feel loved and feel that I should give
love." She became part of a group who prayed over a girl
with multiple sclerosis who couldn't talk, move, or swallow.
Bess concealed her own affliction, determined to get up and
down the stairs without help.

She took over one of the most arduous parts of her son's
paper route seven days a week. After a year, she was able to
think for herself as well, not sick. To her children she was a
normal mother; they helped her just as unwillingly as other chil-

dren do their mothers. Today, in middle age, she walks without a cane and her face shows no wrinkles.

"I had been brought up to think that if you're sick you go to the doctor, not to the Lord. But I think I would have wound up in a wheelchair if I hadn't changed with the Lord's help."

Mildred Smith meditates night and morning with her minister son. He keeps her faith renewed; keeps her believing in herself. He gives her hope. "When I don't get along well, I say, 'I'll do all right tomorrow.' I keep going on that day-to-day faith." She prays each night that she will benefit from her exercises.

"I have faith that God will answer my prayers but I've got to help myself." She doesn't ask for "a miracle," she says. "I have faith that God will give me strength to help myself." She moved from wheelchair to walker and then to the exercise mat at our yoga class. She told me, "I'm just grateful to God that I'm no worse and that I can help myself and I will help myself."

Anne Jackson, a minister's daughter, can still smile with warmth and love despite a series of tragedies—not only her own illness but the death of her fiancé two days after onset of her severe symptoms. She says simply, "I ask God to make everything possible for me." It is, she says, "a hard disease to cope with unless you have faith." In and out of a wheelchair and now on an Amigo, she helps others deal with their problems. In her apartment building, she discovered a woman housebound with multiple sclerosis. She introduced her to the Multiple Sclerosis Society, told her how to apply for Social Security disability benefits, and tried to ignore the woman's dour warning, "You're going to be just like me someday."

The source of her own strength is God. After near death, "from that moment on, I have felt God walks with me and would never abandon me." When she reaches her point of no return, she prays for help. "By believing God can make a way, it just becomes reality."

Brenetta Payne leans a lot on her faith. When she fell in the middle of the street in front of moving cars she prayed to escape being hurt and the cars swerved away. After six years on the job she was fired solely for having multiple sclerosis despite a no-absence record. Worry over the firing triggered an attack of multiple sclerosis because she had a teen-aged daughter to raise with no support from her divorced husband. Finally, she found a good job and continued to practice her religion in the church in her prayer group, outside of church, in befriending the newly diagnosed and others who try to pretend the disease does not exist. She convinced Jewell Phillips to use a cane and told her to "stare back" if anyone stares at her.

Barbara McGrath used to run to early mass with a raincoat over her nightgown to be sure not to miss services. She has remained close to her church. "A lot of people accuse me of using the church as a crutch. I ask, what better crutch can I have?" When her small son, George, told her he didn't believe in God because God hadn't cured her, she responded by saying that God is so busy helping her make cakes for his birthdays, keep him in fresh clothes, and cook for the family that "He doesn't have time to cure me. He's just keeping me well."

I saw the effect faith has had on Dorothy Cox. When I first met her, she had recently joined the charismatic community after abandoning the church for twenty years. A year later, her voice sounded stronger and her words more definite. She seemed more certain of herself. "My faith has deepened very much," she said. "These people have no fears, no worries about the future because their faith in God is strong enough." She acknowledged it was hard to keep the faith; she needs constant reinforcement from others who have faith and from reading the Bible. She sees that others who are worse off than she have no worry for the future. "This doesn't mean that I will be healed but I will be able to live with my handicap at peace and without fear." Instead of resentment and bitterness, she is happy "for the most part." Her life, she says, is "miserable" but *she* isn't.

Dr. Howard Rusk, the authority on rehabilitation who gave Dr. Joseph Panzarella his chance to become the champion of the handicapped, has spoken of the "depth of spirit" of the disabled.

"Fine china," Dr. Rusk said, "doesn't come by putting clay out in the sun to dry. To become china, the clay must go through the white heat of the kiln. In the firing process, some pieces are broken but those that come through are no longer clay but porcelain. So it is with those who have been through the kiln of human experience."

One man I knew could have been broken in the kiln but managed to survive by his stubborn refusal to quit. He was thirty-four years old and a government auditor when he was forced to retire on disability. Within two more years, he was totally helpless, confined to bed, his eyes showing only vague images, his hands shaking, his speech garbled. After fourteen months in the hospital, he had regained some use of one leg and one arm—enough to be released to a nursing home. He was determined to get out of there, too.

He watched his diet, guarded against fatigue, and began to teach himself as a child is taught. He practiced saying words until he could even manage "Methodist Episcopal" with no tongue twisting. He made lines up and down and round and round as a child learns to write. He practiced his ABCs until he could keep even his Rs from going the wrong way. He would try to squeeze a piece of paper into a ball. He was determined to strike a match and kept at it until he finally made it—in his pride ignoring the burns on his fingers.

He had to learn how to turn over in bed, and then relearn

to walk, using two canes. In the course of years, he managed to go slowly up and down stairs. Anything, no matter how difficult, he now tries to do himself, figuring that the more others do for him, the less he will do. As he approaches seventy, he attributes his success—a small business he owns, a car he still drives himself, and his girl friend—to his supreme confidence. "I'm not accustomed to losing."

The secret is to think positively and never give up. In one multiple sclerosis manual I read, a woman said her doctor told her she can do whatever she thinks she can do. She tries anything at least once. But I could tell her that she may have to try some things more than once, even more than a thousand times.

For eleven years, every morning, wherever I was, however I felt, I tried to do sit-ups, but I could never sit up without hooking my feet under a heavy hassock. I tried to strengthen whatever muscles I lacked by crossing my arms over my chest and sitting up without the added push of my arms. But I still had to keep my feet hooked under the hassock. In yoga class, someone had to hold down my feet so I could sit up. It was very embarrassing. Then, one day, after all those years, I sat up without help. After the victory, I was sure I could do anything.

Jean Urciolo told me she tries to achieve one thing a day. On her own, alone in the house, she risked the dizzy heights of standing on a chair to take down the curtains to be washed. She made it without falling, another milestone passed. Maybe you think these are small things—my sit-ups, Jean's curtains—but they are memorable to us.

Jean's husband, John Urciolo, recalled that he used to go to the kitchen to help her bring plates into the dining room. These days, she comes in with them herself. She can get them from the counter to the table. That's a big thing.

"I'm not able to get the lobster meat out of the lobster,"

Jean reminded him, "but I'm working on it. I think if you're grateful for the little things, the big things will come later."

Every day her husband would come home to learn that she had met a new challenge. He used to tease her by wishing aloud that they could harness and use the energy of her trembling arm. "You always could laugh about it. I think that's important."

It was the first time I heard any mention of laughter, but others agreed, when I talked to them later, that being able to laugh—rather than cry—over flailing arms or an unpredictable bladder put such embarrassments in perspective.

Sometimes it may be better not to know the extent of a challenge. I for one would never have embarked on a four-mile walk if I had known that a stroll through the azaleas and camellias and tulips of Mobile's Bellingrath Gardens was that far. At the start, my hostess eyed my cane and asked me if I'd like a wheelchair. Certainly not, I protested. We strolled and strolled, climbing rock steps, negotiating uneven paths. Around me was beauty. And it was as far to go back as to go forward. The endurance test was worthwhile.

Dr. Kathleen Shanahan Cohen believes motivation is significant in managing the disease. The men and women she has seen who are least "aggressive" in improving have nothing they think worth doing. She cited women with multiple sclerosis whose husbands make a reasonably good living, who have no children or whose children are grown, who are not involved in any organization, who do little but eat. She mentioned one woman, once beautiful, now weighing well over two hundred pounds, blaming it all on multiple sclerosis.

Anne Jackson has a great deal that she wants to do and she vows "to fight with the last ounce of my strength." Nothing can stop her, she says. "As long as my brain is functioning, the rest will function. All I have to do is figure out different ways to do things." Her mother had insisted that her children should be positive thinkers. Anne is convinced—and so am I—that positive thoughts actually bring physical benefits. Her neurologist has confirmed that belief.

Frank Uhlmann wholly agrees. During nearly two decades he has seen the humorous side of his illness. Whenever a person gives up, he says, the disease progresses or the body deteriorates much more quickly than it otherwise would. "I say that as a layman rather than a physician, but as one who has done a lot of research on MS and dealt with many individuals who have it."

A friend of Lori Sanjiau's, also with multiple sclerosis, encouraged her to "live each day at a time." He counseled her, "Instead of saying 'my leg is getting weaker, it may be worse tomorrow,' say 'Well I need more work on that leg.'" When Lori met him, he showed no sign of ever having had multiple sclerosis, but when the disease struck, he told her, he had become almost wholly incapacitated. He could not breathe without a respirator; he had lost his vision; he had trouble swallowing; and he could not walk. When his disease went into remission six years ago, he swam every day to strengthen atrophied muscles; he left the safety of his government job to do what he had always wanted to do—go on the road as a Shakespearean actor. Now in his late thirties, he reports that the one carry-over from his attack of multiple sclerosis is a sense of euphoria. "God's way to help someone cope with the disease."

If anyone could be pulled down by the disease, it would be Robert Clark. When I first met him, he had been retired on disability several years from his school building manager's job, but he told me he had come out of this wheelchair twice and would do it a third time. "I'm captain of my ship and my ship still sails," he said confidently. "I've got God's willpower and my own." His goal was to attend his five children's graduations, not in a wheelchair, and to walk down the aisle with his daughters when they grew up and got married.

The next time we talked, he made no mention of leaving the wheelchair. Instead, reacting to a meeting of the President's Committee on Employment of the Handicapped, he said, "Until I saw people with arms and legs off or cerebral palsy I never realized how wonderful it is to see, learn, breathe, talk." Multiple sclerosis seemed such a minor problem compared to what others have.

When I called months later he was in the hospital again. The day he got home he admitted he could no longer get from his wheelchair to a regular chair or into bed without help. Yet he said, of those who pity him, "*You* know how you feel. If you feel stronger, you know it." He assured me that he felt fine.

Sometimes a positive attitude is reflected as much in reaching out to help others as in keeping yourself on the track. John Kramer, the former supersalesman, knows his strength lies in working with others, so he tours the area recommending Amigos and other aids for living to the handicapped. Often, he finds them housebound and depressed, lacking either the information or the imagination to get up again once they have been knocked down.

With his easy laughter, his primer of what is available to them, his tips on where they can go for half-price theater seats, what shopping malls and restaurants they can use, and an Amigo to get there, Kramer can lift the spirits of the most depressed as well as his own. Kramer is one of those who agrees with me that if you have an up attitude and stay busy, you can even retard the progress of the disease.

Not content with a more than full-time job himself and with helping anyone referred to him, Gerry Shur is busy with hobbies. He believes people with multiple sclerosis should develop hobbies that can keep them interested when they can no longer run around. One day, he bought tools to build a dollhouse for his granddaughter. He has never built anything before and says his granddaughter may be beyond the doll stage when he finishes it—"but it will be important while I'm doing it."

Either you live with multiple sclerosis or you don't, Shur says. "You don't have the alternative of getting rid of it. You don't have the alternative of curing it—at least not yet. You do have the alternative of enjoying as much of your life as you can." Thus the dollhouse, the mountain climbing and rock scrambling with his wife, the helping others.

The urgent desire to help others seems to surface in every person who takes a positive attitude toward his multiple sclerosis. Robert Clark told me one of his goals is to teach others how to deal with the disease. Alma Gaghan took the time to drive the man whose multiple sclerosis first terrified her to the Multiple Sclerosis Society to pick up the literature that would help him understand his own disease. Donna Matzureff drives out of her way to take fellow students to Savitri's multiple sclerosis yoga class, although she has a ninety-minute drive each way.

Jeane Hofheimer has turned the golf she loved as a champion into a money-maker for multiple sclerosis. She began to arrange golf tournaments—women's tournaments, because more women than men get multiple sclerosis. The first year she raised $200, the second year $700, the third year $1,500 and she refuses to stop until every golf club in the Washington-Maryland region is committed to holding a tournament for multiple sclerosis.

Golf is only half her double life after she saw her children married (and managed to walk down the aisle each time—the first time alone, the second time with a son to hold on to, the third time between two sons). The other half of her life of helping others is sweaters. She has gathered around her a corps of women who knit. In the eight years of her sweater project, her knitting corps has turned out 4,300 sweaters and 4,200 caps for needy youngsters. Her modus operandi is to assemble and buy the knitting materials and instructions and store them at her apartment house reception desk for her volunteer knitters to collect. There they also leave the completed outfits for Jeane to keep until school opens.

She met many of her knitters for the first time when she received a Community Participation Award from the Washington, D.C., Council on Clothing for Kids. She makes sure that the children of financially pressed victims of multiple sclerosis get the brightly colored knitted outfits, too. "I used to be a sweater girl," Jeane said with a smile. "Now they call me the Sweater Lady."

Jeane lives in my apartment complex, and on summer days I see her sitting outside in the sun. If she longs, as she must, to be on the golf course instead of chatting with old ladies in wheelchairs around the apartment entrance, she never mentions it. She talks enthusiastically about the Redskins' chances in the coming season.

Jeane's unquenchable enthusiasm was one reason I became convinced that helping others can do more than anything else to keep us alive and alert despite whatever physically pulls us down.

For Robert Douglas, whose multiple sclerosis–interrupted life took on new meaning when he taught handicapped youngsters to ride, helping others keeps pain at bay. No matter how busy he is, he finds time to talk to young fellow victims at rap sessions. "Every day is a new day. I find new ways to help people. You've got to welcome all change." The many changes in his own life are "beautiful," he says.

He does not add that while at that moment he can stand the pain, for several nights before he twisted and turned all night in agony.

When after one rap session, I told Douglas that his words

helped these young victims, he responded that it did him good also. "I might be helping others but I'm helping me, too. I don't have time to think about myself."

John R. Brown of New Zealand has traveled thirty thousand miles—much of it in a wheelchair—to help others. Brown had been a school-teaching soccer coach before he began to fall and suffer dizzy spells. When the cause was finally pinned down, his wife left him and he left teaching. But as he could use his hands, his eyes, and his voice, he decided he could be a journalist. So he became education editor of *The Press* in Christchurch. He journeyed to the other side of the world as a Winston Churchill Memorial Trust Traveling Fellow, picking up a wheelchair in London. When I met him at a multiple sclerosis conference in Washington, he was on the way home with more than a hundred and fifty hours of tape recordings of his experiences. As a former athlete himself, he was impressed by the athletes who are raising funds for multiple sclerosis in the Athletes *vs.* MS program, which he called "the finest example I've seen of the healthy helping the disabled."

Faith and resolve have carried him a long way. "I pray a lot. I pray that I will have time in my life to give the knowledge I have gained and the hope I have gained to others with the disease." He hopes his thirty-thousand-mile trip will give others hope.

Helping others has become the goal, the avocation, the hobby, even the career of many people with multiple sclerosis. Typical of them is Steve Drakulich, former chairman and patient services director of the Nevada Central Chapter of the Multiple Sclerosis Society in Reno and now a board member and its leading fund-raiser. His disease was discovered in the air force during World War II. He has been in a wheelchair since 1965 but the governor of his state has praised him as "a man who can't be beaten and won't be beaten." He distributes wheelchairs, arranges for visiting nurses and home-makers, counsels the newly diagnosed, and conducts a variety of fund-raising events from barbecues to ballets. His wife, who is his chauffeur and as involved as he in patient problems, says if he wasn't in a wheelchair she could never keep up with him.

When a physician calls him to the hospital to talk to new patients, he tries to counter their depression. "It helps for me to tell them that I've had the damn disease for over thirty years. They perk right up when they see me and hear that." It gives him "a good feeling."

That "good feeling," that impulse to help others, must have some good physical effect because even those usually considered selfish and egocentric seem to warm to the idea of doing something for somebody else. It is almost as if they feel instinctively that the milk of human kindness could nourish them. You may not actually *be* better, but you *feel* better.

There are dozens of ways to help others if you are a victim yourself. You can answer questions for multiple sclerosis researchers. You can make sure that children in your schools join the MS READ-a-thon to raise funds for multiple sclerosis by getting neighbors to pledge a sum for every book they read. You can use your own know-how to advise fellow patients how to live with this disorder.

Dr. Shanahan Cohen suggested another method of benefiting both giver and receiver when I asked her what she thought would most help people, short of a cure.

"An opportunity to talk about it," she promptly replied. "What they really need is an MS Anonymous. So when you're climbing walls there's somebody you have established a relationship with, someone you can call and say, 'I'm going out of my mind. I wasn't able to button my shirt sleeves this morning.' This is the sort of thing that can panic people, make them think they are having an exacerbation. It would help tremendously if they could call someone who could tell them they, too, frequently have trouble with buttons, and that they're not having an exacerbation, it's just that their coordination isn't so good today. The blouse may be beautiful, but save it for a day when they're feeling great."

An MS Anonymous, she said, would give those with the disease a chance to talk to one another, and, I contend, in that interchange both the caller and the called would benefit physically as well as emotionally or mentally.

Until research finds a cure, this is as far as my pursuit of hope can go. I think it's a long way. We have found—most of us—that with faith in God, faith in our own positive thoughts, and a willingness, even an eagerness, to help others, we can live with this thing and live well.

Index